Infrared Imaging

A casebook in clinical medicine

Infrared Imaging

A casebook in clinical medicine

Francis Ring
University of South Wales, UK

Anna Jung
Military Institute of Medicine, Poland

Janusz Żuber
Military Institute of Medicine, Poland

IOP Publishing, Bristol, UK

ISBN 978-0-7503-1143-4 (ebook)
ISBN 978-0-7503-1144-1 (print)
ISBN 978-0-7503-1145-8 (mobi)

DOI 10.1088/978-0-7503-1143-4

Version: 20150801

IOP Expanding Physics
ISSN 2053-2563 (online)
ISSN 2054-7315 (print)

British Library Cataloguing-in-Publication Data: A catalogue record for this book is available from the British Library.

Published by IOP Publishing, wholly owned by The Institute of Physics, London

IOP Publishing, Temple Circus, Temple Way, Bristol, BS1 6HG, UK

US Office: IOP Publishing, Inc., 190 North Independence Mall West, Suite 601, Philadelphia, PA 19106, USA

Dedicated to the late Baron Professor Leopold Thibault de Boesinghe MD of Gent University Belgium, a pioneer in medical thermography and former President of the European Association of Thermology.

Contents

Part 4 The upper extremities

Preface

Twelve years ago, Anna Jung, Janusz Zuber and Francis Ring edited the *Casebook of Infrared Imaging in Clinical Medicine* with text in Polish and English for MedPress in Poland.

Great progress has since been made in both infrared camera techniques and the understanding of the significance of infrared imaging in clinical medicine. Whilst this new book contains about a third of the chapters from the original casebook, it now provides significantly more than a simple update of the field. In addition to including many new case reports signaling the importance and extension of clinical medical infrared imaging, the theoretical section has been extended with significant papers, some previously published in journals, that provide a framework for recording, evaluating and interpreting infrared thermal images in clinical medicine.

The order of chapters follows the anatomical regions and is not a catalogue of diseases. In this way it makes clear that variations in the level and distribution of temperature are not a 'signature of disease', but a strong indicator of disease or physiologic activity. As heat radiation is mostly determined by blood flow in the superficial skin vasculature, and blood flow itself is dependent on the portion of cardiac output, the density of blood vessels and the width of the vascular bed, wider and more vessels will result in higher blood flow leading to more heat radiation which is coded as higher temperature in infrared thermal images. Such an increase of temperature might be the result of inflammation, newly built vessels or simply of vasodilation due to an effector response of the thermoregulation system.

Under well controlled environmental conditions and patient preparation, thermoregulation responses can be avoided, and in patients with an established diagnosis the course of temperature recorded in a lesion with infrared imaging reflects the activity of the underlying disease. Areas of low skin temperature indicate reduced blood flow and the course of temperature after applying a cold stimulus can differentiate short lasting episodes of vasoconstriction from severe vasospasms or poor perfusion due to occluded vessels.

This new casebook provides good examples of the value of infrared imaging as an outcome measure in clinical medicine.

Professor Kurt Ammer MD, PhD

Acknowledgements

The editors wish to thank all the contributing authors to this book—the clinical colleagues and members of the European Association of Thermology who have provided images and case reports. This has resulted in a widespread record of clinical experience with this technology of infrared thermal imaging. Not all submitted material could be included, so we thank all those colleagues who supplied material for this particular project. There are also some published papers that have been in particular demand since their original publication. We therefore express thanks to the journals that have given permission for these selected papers to be reproduced. To Medpress in Warsaw we express our thanks for the cases selected for inclusion from the earlier shorter Casebook published over a decade ago. Some earlier papers included indicate that the quality of the thermographic images has dramatically improved over recent years, due to significant improvements in the technology. We thank those manufacturers who have assisted in the clinical studies, especially where excellent high resolution images have been obtained.

About the editors

Francis Ring

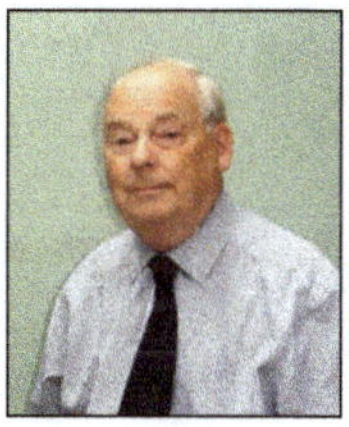

Francis Ring has worked for over 50 years with infrared thermography in medicine. He is currently Director of The Medical Imaging Research Unit at The University of South Wales in the United Kingdom. He holds a medal awarded by The Combined Colleges (Medicine, Surgery and Gynaecology in the UK) for his lifetime research into medical applications of infrared imaging.

Anna Jung

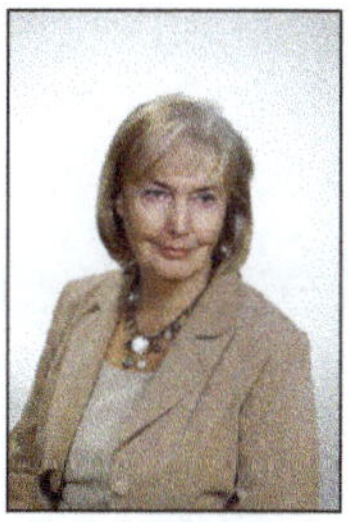

Anna Jung, is Professor of Pediatrics with a DSc in Medical Sciences at the Central Clinical Hospital of Military Institute of Medicine in Warsaw, Poland. Professor Jung has worked for over 20 years with infrared thermography in medicine and conducts studies, supported by the State Committee for Scientific Research, on the application of thermographic methods in medical diagnostics.

She was awarded the Knight's Cross of the Order of Polonia Restituta by the President of Poland for her achievements in the fields of medical science.

Janusz Żuber

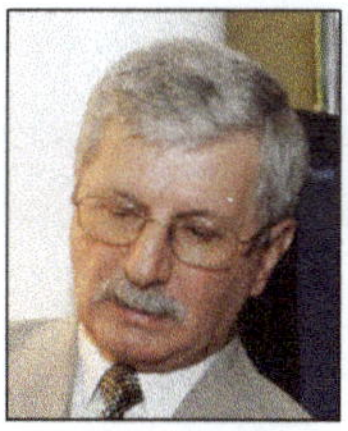

Janusz Żuber, MD PhD has experience of over 20 years in the Clinical Thermography of the Central Clinical Hospital of Military Institute of Medicine in Warsaw, Poland. He is the author of numerous works on the application of liquid crystal thermography and thermal imaging in allergic medicine and other applications in medical diagnostics.

List of contributors

John Allen
Microvascular Diagnostics
Regional Medical Physics Department
The Newcastle upon Tyne Hospitals NHS Foundation Trust
Newcastle upon Tyne
UK
and
Institute of Cellular Medicine
Newcastle University
Newcastle upon Tyne
UK

Kurt Ammer
European Association of Thermography
Vienna
Austria
and
Medical Imaging Research Unit
Faculty of Mathematics, Computing and Science
University of South Wales
Pontypridd
Wales
UK

K Bilska
Department of Oncological Surgery of Children and Adolescents
Mother and Child Institute
Warsaw
Poland

Stephen Burnett
Microvascular Diagnostics
Regional Medical Physics Department
The Newcastle upon Tyne Hospitals NHS Foundation Trust
Newcastle upon Tyne
UK

Rui Carvalho
Diabetic Foot Clinic
Centro Hospitalar do Porto EPE
Porto
Portugal

Mirosław Dąbrowski
Institute of Optoelectronics
Military University of Technology
Warsaw
Poland

Costanzo Di Maria
Microvascular Diagnostics
Regional Medical Physics Department
The Newcastle upon Tyne Hospitals NHS Foundation Trust
Newcastle upon Tyne
UK
and
Institute of Cellular Medicine
Newcastle University
Newcastle upon Tyne
UK

Jane Dickinson
Department of Ophthalmology
The Newcastle upon Tyne Hospitals NHS Foundation Trust
Newcastle upon Tyne
UK

Ana Domingues
Faculty of Engineering
University of Porto
Porto
Portugal

Rafał Dulski
Institute of Optoelectronics
Military University of Technology
Warsaw
Poland

Liliana Esteves
Faculty of Engineering
University of Porto
Porto
Portugal

V Flower
The Royal National Hospital for Rheumatic Diseases
Bath
UK

Ian Forrest
Musculoskeletal Unit
The Newcastle upon Tyne Hospitals NHS Foundation Trust
Newcastle upon Tyne
UK

Joaquim Gabriel
LABIOMEP, INEGI
Faculty of Engineering
University of Porto
Porto
Portugal

Z Gacion
Clinic of Internal Diseases, Hypertension and Angiology
Medical University of Warsaw
Warsaw
Poland

Ł Gadomska vel Betka
Clinic of Internal Diseases, Hypertension and Angiology
Medical University of Warsaw
Warsaw
Poland

Lech Gawron
Ophthalmology Clinic
Department of Pediatrics, Pediatric Nephrology and Allergology
Military Institute of Medicine
Warsaw
Poland

Grainne Gorman
Department of Neurology
Royal Victoria Infirmary
The Newcastle upon Tyne Hospitals NHS Foundation Trust
Newcastle upon Tyne
UK
and
Wellcome Trust Centre for Mitochondrial Research
Institute of Neuroscience
Newcastle University
Newcastle upon Tyne
UK

Ryszard Grenda
Nephrology Clinic Institute
Pomnik – Centrum Zdrowia Dziecka
Warsaw
Poland

Bridget Griffiths
Institute of Cellular Medicine
Medical School
Newcastle University
Newcastle upon Tyne
UK

D Hart
Department of Clinical Measurement
The Royal National Hospital for Rheumatic Diseases
Bath
UK

Katarzyna Jobs
Department of Pediatrics, Pediatric Nephrology and Allergology
Military Institute of Medicine
Warsaw
Poland

Anna Jung
Department of Pediatrics, Pediatric Nephrology and Allergology
Military Institute of Medicine
Warsaw
Poland

Bolesław Kalicki
Department of Pediatrics, Pediatric Nephrology and Allergology
Military Institute of Medicine
Warsaw
Poland

Marek Klewar
Radiology Department
Military School of Medicine
Warsaw
Poland

Jakub Klimkiewicz
Department of Anesthesiology and Intensive Care
Military Institute of Medicine
Warsaw
Poland

A Koszycka
Thermal Laboratory of Pediatric, Nephrology and Allergology Clinic
Military Institute of Medicine
Warsaw
Poland

A Krawczyk
ICT Department
Military Institute of Medicine
Warsaw
Poland

Rafał Kuligowski
Department of Pediatrics, Pediatric Nephrology and Allergology
Military Institute of Medicine
Warsaw
Poland

Nicola Leech
Newcastle Diabetes Centre
Centre for Ageing and Vitality
The Newcastle upon Tyne Hospitals NHS Foundation Trust
Newcastle uopn Tyne
UK

Aleksander Ligęziński
ENT Department Clinic
Central Hospital
Military School of Medicine
Warsaw
Poland

A Lipińska-Opałka
Department of Pediatrics, Pediatric Nephrology and Allergology
Military Institute of Medicine
Warsaw
Poland

Weronika Machura
Department of Anesthesiology and Intensive Care
Military Institute of Medicine
Warsaw
Poland

Ana Marques
Faculty of Engineering
University of Porto
Porto
Portugal

Marcin Możański
Department of Anesthesiology and Intensive Care
Military Institute of Medicine
Warsaw
Poland

J Mróz
Rehabilitation Clinic
Military Institute of Medicine
Warsaw
Poland

Piotr Murawski
ICT Department
Military Institute of Medicine
Warsaw
Poland

B Nurowska-Wrzosek
Clinic of Internal Diseases, Hypertension and Angiology
Medical University of Warsaw
Warsaw
Poland

Crispian Oates
Vascular Ultrasound
Department of Radiology
The Newcastle upon Tyne Hospitals NHS Foundation Trust
Newcastle upon Tyne
UK

João Oliveira
Faculty of Medicine
University of Porto
Porto
Portugal

Michał Osiecki
Radiology Department
Central Hospital
Military School of Medicine
Warsaw
Poland

J D Pauling
The Royal National Hospital for Rheumatic Diseases
Bath
UK

Wojciech Perdzyński
Department of Children Surgery
Central Hospital
Military School of Medicine
Warsaw
Poland

Petros Perros
Institute of Genetic Medicine
Newcastle University
Newcastle upon Tyne
UK

Madalena Pimenta
Department of Radiology
Hospital de São João
Porto
Portugal

Cezary Pogorzelski
Dentistry Institute
Central Clinical Hospital
Military Medical Academy
Warsaw
Poland

Marco Rebelo
Plastic and Reconstructive Surgery Service
IPO-Porto
Porto
Portugal

E F J Ring
Medical Imaging Research Unit
Faculty of Mathematics, Computing and Science
University of South Wales
Pontypridd
Wales
UK

Derek Robertshaw
Newcastle Diabetes Centre
Centre for Ageing and Vitality
The Newcastle upon Tyne Hospitals NHS Foundation Trust
Newcastle uopn Tyne
UK

Radosław Różycki
Ophthalmology Clinic
Department of Pediatrics, Pediatric Nephrology and Allergology
Military Institute of Medicine
Warsaw
Poland

A Rustecka
Department of Pediatrics, Pediatric Nephrology and Allergology
Military Institute of Medicine
Warsaw
Poland

Bartosz Rustecki
Department of Anesthesiology and Intensive Care
Military Institute of Medicine
Warsaw
Poland

J Shipley
Department of Clinical Measurement
The Royal National Hospital for Rheumatic Diseases
Bath
UK

Marek Stańczyk
II Surgery Department
Central Hospital
Military School of Medicine
Warsaw
Poland

W Stankiewicz
Military Institute of Hygiene and Epidemiology
Warsaw
Poland

Andrzej Stankiewicz
Ophthalmology Clinic
Department of Pediatrics, Pediatric Nephrology and Allergology
Military Institute of Medicine
Warsaw
Poland

David Talbot
Renal Medicine and Transplant Centre
The Newcastle upon Tyne Hospitals NHS Foundation Trust
Newcastle upon Tyne
UK

João Torres
Faculty of Medicine
University of Porto
Porto
Portugal
and
Department of Orthopaedics
Hospital de São João
Porto
Portugal

Paweł Twarkowski
Radiology Department
Central Hospital
Military School of Medicine
Warsaw
Poland

Ricardo Vardasca
LABIOMEP, INEGI
Faculty of Engineering
University of Porto
Porto
Portugal
and
Medical Imaging Research Unit
Faculty of Mathematics, Computing and Science
University of South Wales
Pontypridd
Wales

W Woźniak
Department of Oncological Surgery of Children and Adolescents
Mother and Child Institute
Warsaw
Poland

Paweł Zaborowski
Dentistry Institute
Central Clinical Hospital
Military Medical Academy
Warsaw
Poland

Stanisław Żmuda
Dentistry Institute
Military Medical Academy
Warsaw
Poland

Janusz Żuber
Department of Pediatrics, Pediatric Nephrology and Allergology
Military Institute of Medicine
Warsaw
Poland

Chapter 1

The technique of infrared imaging in medicine*

1.1 Introduction

Infrared thermal imaging has been used in medicine since the early 1960s. Early imaging systems were large with very limited facilities for display and temperature measurement. In the 1970s computer image processing of thermograms became available, with increased possibilities for quantitation and archiving of images [1]. This resulted in an increased awareness of the need for standardization of techniques. Two publications were initiated by working groups within the European Thermographic Association (now European Association of Thermology) to address this question. The first, 'Standardisation of thermography in locomotor diseases—recommended procedure' [2], set out the basic requirements for techniques agreed by a European panel of rheumatologists and radiologists. This paper, which was published in 1978, contained many elements of standardization which applied to other clinical applications of thermography. The second, 'Skin temperature measurement in drug trials' [3], was presented by a group of authors who described the essential techniques for the use of thermography in clinical drug trials. The proceedings of a special conference on breast diseases published in 1983 included a chapter on the 'Standardisation of thermal imaging: physical and environmental influences' [4]. A further statement from the European Association of Thermology was published in 1988 on the subject of 'Raynaud's phenomenon: assessment by thermography' [5]. An overview of recommendations gathered from The American Academy of Thermology, The Japanese Society of Biomedical Thermology and the European Association of Thermology was collated and published by Clark *et al* in 1997 [6]. This paper is based on the practical implications of the previous papers taken from the perspective of the modern thermal imaging systems available to medicine.

*First published in Ring E F J and Ammer K 2000 *Thermol. Int.* **10** 7–14.

doi:10.1088/978-0-7503-1143-4ch1

1.2 Location for thermal imaging

1.2.1 Investigation room

The room used for thermal imaging must meet certain basic requirements. These are: adequate size for working— where up to 2 m may be needed between the patient and the subject—and adequate space to locate the image processing equipment and space for one or more patient cubicles. A rough indicator for the least distance in one direction can be derived from the optical features of the lens, i.e. the distance between the camera and the patient to take an image of the upper or lower part of the human body or of an object of 1.2 m height. This means that a minimum size of 2 m × 3 m is required, but that a larger room, 3 m × 4 m or more, is preferable.

1.2.2 Ambient temperature control

This is a primary requirement for most clinical applications of thermal imaging. A range of temperatures from 18 °C to 25 °C should be attainable and held for at least 1 h at an accuracy better than 1 °C. At lower temperatures the subject is likely to shiver and an over 25 °C room temperature will cause sweating, at least in most European countries. Variations may be expected in colder or warmer climates, in the latter case, room temperatures may need to be 1–2 °C higher [7].

The type of examination used will determine the ideal ambient temperature. Many clinical examinations are performed with partial disrobing of the patient. When larger areas of the body are unclothed and exposed to the air for longer periods, lower ambient temperatures will cause discomfort [8, 9] and may result in reflex vasoconstriction. Inflammatory lesions are more clearly visualized in a cool environment, typically 20 °C. Examination of the extremities, where the sympathetic nervous system influences the result, a warmer ambient temperature of 22–24 °C is generally recommended.

Additional techniques for cooling particular regions of the body have been developed [10, 11] (e.g. water immersion of the hands in a stress test).

1.2.3 Room temperature indication

Indication of the air temperature is important, a large digital display which is visible anywhere in the room should be used. Air temperature is affected not only by the heat generated by electronic equipment, but also by the human body. For this reason the air-conditioning unit should be capable of compensating for the maximum number of patients and staff likely to be in the room at any one time. These effects will be greater in a small room of 2 m × 3 m or less. Air-conditioning equipment should be located so that direct draughts are not directed at the patient and that overall air speed is kept as low as possible. A suspended perforated ceiling with ducts diffusing the air distribution evenly over the room is ideal [12], although more expensive to construct, than simple wall mounted systems.

1.2.4 Computer and other equipment

Image processing equipment needs space located away from the patient area, to avoid heat disturbance. A sink with a water supply is often required for water stress tests.

Furniture may also include a multi-position chair with attached leg rests and a bowl or table on castors at a suitable height for a sitting patient.

1.2.5 Patient cubicle

Finally a cubicle or cubicles within the temperature controlled area are essential. These should provide privacy for disrobing and a suitable area for resting through the acclimatization period.

1.3 The imaging system

1.3.1 The camera system

A new generation of infrared cameras have become available for medical imaging. The older systems, normally single-element detectors using an optical mechanical scanning process, were mostly cooled by the addition of liquid nitrogen [13–15]. This had the effect of limiting the angle at which the camera could be used, which restricted operation. Electronic cooling systems were then introduced, which overcame this problem. The latest generation of focal plane array cameras can be used without cooling, providing almost maintenance-free technology [16].

Almost all systems now use image processing techniques and provide basic quantitation of the image [17–19]. In some cases this may be operated from a chip within the camera, or may be carried out through an on-line or off-line computer. For older equipment such as the AGA 680 series, several hardware adaptations have been reported to achieve quantitation of the thermograms [20–22].

1.3.2 Temperature reference

Earlier reports stipulated the requirement for a separate thermal reference source for calibration checks on the camera [23]. Many systems now include an internal reference temperature, with manufacturers claiming that external checks are not required. Unless frequent servicing is obtained, it is still advisable to use an external source, if only to check for drift in the temperature sensitivity of the camera. An external reference, which may be purchased or constructed, can be switched on with the equipment and left running throughout the day. This allows the operator to make checks on the camera and, in particular, provides a check on the hardware and software employed for processing. These constant temperature source checks may be the only satisfactory way of proving the reliability of temperature measurements made from the thermogram [24].

1.3.3 Mounting the imager

A camera stand which provides vertical height adjustment is very important for medical thermography. Photographic tripod stands are inconvenient for frequent adjustments and often result in tilting the camera at an undefined angle to the patient. This is difficult to reproduce and, unless the patient is positioned so that the surface scanned is aligned at 90° to the camera lens, distortion of the image is unavoidable. Studio camera stands are ideal, they provide vertical height adjustment with counterbalance weight compensation. They are stable with a weighted base on wheels which enables the operator to rapidly set up the camera in any reproducible position. Most stands can hold the camera to within 10 cm from the floor (the patient can also stand on a low stool to avoid parallax even in a standing position). The maximum height required will depend on the use of a low couch, or whether all positioning is achieved with the patient standing or sitting in a chair. A pillar height of 2 m or 2.5 m can be used. It should be noted that the type of lens used on the camera will affect the working distance and the field of view, a wide angle lens reduces distance between the camera and the subject in many cases, but may also increase peripheral distortion of the image. The ceiling mounted stands used in radiology and nuclear medicine can also be used, but are likely to require positioning motors if the camera is beyond the operators reach.

1.3.4 Camera initialization

The start-up times with modern cameras are claimed to be very short, minutes or seconds. However, the speed with which the image becomes visible is not an indication of image stability. Checks on calibration will usually show that a much longer period from 10 min to several hours with an uncooled system are needed to achieve optimum conditions for quantitative imaging [4, 25].

1.3.5 Image processing

Software packages for thermal imaging are provided by some manufacturers, few of which are specifically designed for medical applications [17, 18]. One specialized software system designed for medical use meets international standards when used according to recommended techniques [26]. Archiving of both images and relevant clinical data is an important requirement for medical thermography.

1.4 The patient

1.4.1 Patient information

Human skin temperature is the product of heat dissipated from the vessels and organs within the body, and the effect of environmental factors on heat loss or gain. There are a number of further influences which are controllable, such as cosmetics [27], alcohol intake [28] and smoking [29–31]. These should form part of the request made to the patient when calling him or her for examination. In general terms the patient attending the examination should be advised to avoid all topical applications such as ointments [32, 33] and cosmetics on the day of the examination to all the relevant areas of the body. Large meals and above-average intake of tea or coffee should also be avoided, although studies supporting this recommendation are hard to find and the results are not conclusive [34–36]. Patients should be asked to avoid tight fitting clothing and to keep physical exertion to a minimum. This particularly applies to methods of physiotherapy such as electrotherapy [37–39], ultrasound [40], heat treatment [41–43], cryotherapy [43–46], massage [47–49] and hydrotherapy [50–52] because the thermal effects from such treatments can last for 4–6 h under certain conditions. Heat production by muscular exercise is a well-documented phenomenon [53–57].

Drug treatments can also affect the skin temperature. This phenomenon was used to evaluate the therapeutic effects of medicaments [3]. Drugs affecting the cardiovascular system [58–61] must be reported to the thermographer in order that the correct interpretation of thermal images will be given.

1.4.2 Pre-imaging equilibration

On arrival at the department, the patient should be informed of the examination procedure, instructed to remove appropriate clothing and jewellery, and asked to sit or rest in the preparation cubicle for a fixed time. The time required to achieve adequate stability in blood pressure and skin temperature is generally considered to be 15 min, with 10 min as a minimum [62–64]. After 30 min of cooling, oscillations of the skin temperature can be detected in different regions of the body with different amplitudes resulting in a temperature asymmetry between the left and right sides [63]. Some evidence has been found for a circadian rhythm of both core and skin temperatures [20, 34, 65, 66]. During this preparation time the patient must avoid folding or crossing their arms or legs, or placing their bare feet on a cold surface. If the lower extremities are to be examined, a stool or leg rest should be provided to avoid direct contact with the floor [67]. During the examination paper or linen towels may be required to avoid overcooling of the feet.

1.4.3 Positions for imaging

As in radiology, it is preferable to standardize on a series of standard views for each body region. The EAT Locomotor Diseases Group recommendations include a triangular marker system to indicate anterior, posterior, lateral and angled views [2, 68]. Modern image processing software provides comment boxes which can be used to encode the angle of view which will be stored with the image [26]. It should be noted that the position of the patient for scanning and in preparation must be constant. Standing, sitting or lying down affects the surface area of the body exposed to the ambient temperature, therefore an image recorded with the patient in a sitting position may not be comparable with one recorded on a separate occasion in a standing position.

1.4.4 Field of view

Image size is dependent on the distance between the camera and the patient and the focal length of the infrared camera lens. The lens is generally fixed on most medical systems, so it is good practice to maintain a constant distance from the patient for each view in order to acquire a reproducible field of view for the image. For example a single hand may be recorded in a 20 cm × 20 cm field of view, while a picture of both lower limbs from knees to ankles may require a 50 cm × 50 cm field. If deviations in camera angle from the normal position on the stand are required, these should be recorded for future use. If different thermograms with different fields are compared for the same subject, the variable resolution can lead to false temperature readings [69]. Most hospitals now use a standard format for patient identification and demographic detail. As much detail as possible should be recorded with the thermogram to avoid misidentification. The time and date of the examination should also be recorded, which most computer software will provide as standard [70].

1.5 Report generation

1.5.1 Colour and temperature scale

Individual software programmes now largely dictate the layout for a clinical report. This will normally consist of the images, the demographic data and any measurements made from image processing. Every image or block of images must carry an indication of temperature range, with colour code/temperature scale. The colour scale itself should be standardized. Industrial software frequently provides a grey-scale picture and one or more colour scales. The default colour scale will often show white as hot, then yellow and then red, following the hot metal scale. The so-called rainbow or spectral order of colours is more widely recognized, especially by colleagues who are not used to the other colour scales used by engineers. A false colour finely graded scale is also possible, this can range from dark blue at the cold end through green to red and will convey a similar degree of image contrast to a monochrome black and white picture.

1.5.2 Processing the reported image

Background temperatures which can obscure the clinical image should be avoided and cleaning the image by processing, e.g. squeezing the temperature range or overwriting the lower temperatures with a background of white, grey or black, will improve the visual presentation. Care should be taken when the pictures are recorded to minimize these problems. The use of hardboard or cold towels arranged just prior to image recording will often improve the image clarity. Regions of interest, spot measurements sites, etc, should be indicated and, if these mask the clinical picture, a separate image without these processing indicators should be provided. It is important to note that while a high number of colour shades can be displayed on a computer monitor screen, most printers to date are less able to reproduce all the fine detail. Settings for the image on the screen should be tested on the printer to ensure that subtle differences in the image which are important are not lost in a lower contrast printed image.

1.5.3 Archiving images and data

Computer file archives are now commonplace and are a valuable reference for repeated investigations on the same patient. A multiple window facility in the software will allow the operator to recall a series of earlier pictures for comparison and to ensure that the same positions and temperature settings have been used. A matrix of 4×4 images is adequate with the possibility to zoom in on any combination of frames for the report [24]. The numerical data relating to each image must be clearly identified with the original image to which they relate. If a standardized challenge test such as a cold stress test for Raynaud's phenomenon has been used, the relevant images should be printed, preferably to show the pre- and post-stress thermograms together with the temperature data extracted from them.

Where normal values for indices [71–73] or temperature values [74, 75] are known, these should be included in the report.

1.6 Conclusion

Good technique is essential with infrared imaging, which is a physiological procedure. Attention to details as described will improve physicians' ability to use the techniques as a diagnostic aid and for monitoring change from treatment or from the natural course of the disease. Good documentation and self-explanatory reports will improve the clinical acceptability of the technique. Such requirements are expected from any imaging procedure used as medico-legal evidence. The same standard should apply to routine clinical investigations with thermal imaging. Poor image reproduction and incomplete reporting will serve to deter clinical use. Few non-invasive imaging techniques are as easily quantified as infrared imaging. The modern equipment available since 1999 is of superior quality and reliability to any previously used in medicine.

References

[1] Ring E F J 1975 Thermography and rheumatic diseases *Bibl. Radiol.* **6** 97–106

[2] Engel J M, Cosh J A, Ring E F J, Page-Thomas D P, Van Waes P and Shoenfeld D 1979 Thermography in locomotor diseases—recommended procedure *Eur. J. Rheumatology Inflammation* **2** 299–306

[3] Ring E F J, Engel J M and Page-Thomas D P 1984 Thermologic methods in clinical pharmacology—skin temperature measurement in drug trials *Int. J. Clin. Pharmacol. Ther. Toxicol.* **22** 20–4

[4] Ring E F J 1983 *Standardisation of Thermal Imaging in Medicine: Physical and Environmental Factors in Thermal Assessment of Breast Health* ed M Gautherie, E Albert and L Keith (Lancaster: MTP) pp 29–36

[5] Aarts N *et al* European Association of Thermology 1988 Raynaud's phenomenon: assessment by thermography *Thermology* **3** 69–73

[6] Clark R P and de Calcina-Goff M 1997 Guidelines for standardisation in medical thermography draft international standard proposals *Thermol. Österreich* **7** 47–58

[7] Ishigaki T, Ikeda M, Asai H and Sakuma S 1989 Forehead-back thermal ratio for the interpretation of infrared imaging of spinal cord lesions and other neurological disorders *Thermology* **3** 101–7

[8] Issing K and Hensel H 1982 Temperaturempfindung und thermischer Komfort bei statischen Temperaturreizen *Z. Phys. Med. Baln Med. Klim.* **11** 354–65

[9] Mabuchi K, Kanbara O, Genno H, Chinzei T, Haeno S and Kunimoto M 1997 Automatic control of optimum ambient thermal conditions using feedback of skin temperature *Biomed. Thermology* **16** 6–13

[10] Schuber T R, d Haute J V, Hassenburger J and Beller F K 1977 Directed dynamic cooling: a methodic contribution in telethermography *Acta Thermographica* **2** 94–9

[11] Di Carlo A 1994 Thermography in patients with systemic sclerosis *Thermol. Österreich* **4** 18–24

[12] Love T J 1985 Heat transfer considerations in the design of a thermology clinic *Thermology* **1** 88–91

[13] Dibley D A G 1995 Opto-mechanical systems for thermal imaging *The Thermal Image in Medicine and Biology* ed K Ammer and E F J Ring (Vienna: Uhlen) pp 33–9

[14] Friedrich K H 1980 Assessment criteria for infrared thermography systems *Acta Thermographica* **5** 68–76

[15] Alderson J K A and Ring E F J 1985 'Sprite' high resolution thermal imaging system *Thermology* **1** 110–14

[16] Kutas M 1984 Staring focal plane array for medical thermal imaging *Recent Advances in Medical Thermology* ed E F J Ring and B Phillips (New York: Plenum) pp 185–94

[17] Engel J M 1983 Thermotom: ein Softwarepaket für die thermographische Bildanalyse in der Rheumatologie *Biomed. Tech.* **26** 115–16

[18] Bösiger P and Scaroni F 1983 Mikroprozessor- unterstütztes Thermographie-System zur quantitativewn on-line Analyse von statischen und dynamischen Thermogrammen *Thermologische Messmethodik* ed J-M Engel, U Flesch and F Stüttgen (Baden-Baden: Notamed) pp 125–30

[19] Brandes P 1994 PIC-Win-Iris Bildverarbeitungssoftware *Thermol. Österreich* **4** 33–5

[20] Ring E F J 1977 Quantitative thermography in arthritis using the AGA integrator *Acta Thermographica* **2** 172–6

[21] Parr G, Prees M, Salisbury R, Page Thomas P and Hazleman B R 1984 Microcomputer standardization of the AGA 680 M system Recent *Advances In Medical Thermology* ed E F J Ring and B Phillips (New York: Plenum) pp 211–14

[22] Van Hamme H, De Geest G and Cornelis J 1990 An acquisition and scan conversion unit for the AGA THV680 medical infrared camera *Thermology* **3** 205–8

[23] Committee on Quality Control and Qualifications of the American Academy of Thermology 1986 Technical Guidelines, Edition 2 *Thermology* **2** 108–12

[24] Ring E F J 1984 Quality control in infrared thermography *Recent Advances In Medical Thermology* ed E F J Ring and B Phillips (New York: Plenum) pp 185–94

[25] Ring E F J, Minchinton M and Elvins D M 1999 A focal plane array system for clinical infrared imaging Ann. Int. Conf. IEEE Engineering in Medicine and Biology Society (13–16 October 1999, Atlanta, GA) paper 11.6.3 p 1120

[26] Plassmann P and Ring E F J 1997 An open system for the acquisition and evaluation of medical thermological images *Eur. J. Thermol.* **7** 216–20

[27] Engel J-M 1984 Physical and physiological influence of medical ointments of infrared thermography *Recent Advances in Medical Thermology* ed E F J Ring and B Phillips (New York: Plenum) pp 177–84

[28] Mannara G, Salvatori G C and Pizzuti G P 1993 Ethyl alcohol induced skin temperature changes evaluated by thermography. Preliminary results *Boll. Soc. Ital. Biol. Sper.* **69** 587–94

[29] Usuki K, Kanekura T, Aradono K and Kanzaki T 1998 Effects of nicotine on peripheral cutaneous blood flow and skin temperature *J. Dermatol. Sci.* **16** 173–81

[30] Gershon-Cohen J and Haberman J 1968 Thermography of smoking *Arch. Environ.* **16** 637–41

[31] Gershon-Cohen J, Borden A G and Hermel M B 1969 Thermography of extremities after smoking *Br. J. Radiol.* **42** 189–91

[32] Hejazi S and Anbar M 1993 Effects of topical skin treatment and of ambient light in infrared thermal images *Biomed. Thermol.* **12** 300–05

[33] Ammer K 1997 The influence of antirheumatic creams and ointments on the infrared emission of the skin *Abs. 10th Int. Conf. Thermogrammetry and Thermal Engineering* 18–20 June 1997, Budapest ed I Benkö *et al* (Budapest: MATE) pp 177–81

[34] Reinberg A 1975 Circadian changes in the temperature of human beings *Bibl. Radiol.* **6** 128–39

[35] Federspil G, La Grassa E, Giordano F, Macor C, Presacco D and Di Maggio C 1989 Study of diet-induced thermogenesis using telethermography in normal and obese subjects *Recenti Prog. Med.* **80** 455–9

[36] Shlygin G K, Lindenbraten L D, Gapparov M M, Vasilevskaia L S, Ginzburg L I and Sokolov A I 1991 Radio- thermometric research of tissues during the initial reflex period of the specific dynamic action of food *Med. Radiol. (Mosk.)* **36** 10–2

[37] Danz J and Callies R 1979 Infrarothermometrie bei differenzierten Methoden der Niederfrequenztherapie *Z. Physiother.* **31** 35–9

[38] Rusch F, Neeck G and Schmidt K L 1988 Über die Hemmung von Erythemen durch Capsaicin. 3. Objektivierung des Capsaicin-Erythems mittels statischer und dynamischer Thermographie *Z. Phys. Med. Baln. Med. Klim.* **17** 18–24

[39] Mayr H, Thür H and Ammer K 1995 Electrical stimulation of the stellate ganglia *The Thermal Image in Medicine and Biology* ed K Ammer and E F J Ring (Vienna: Uhlen) pp 206–9

[40] Danz J and Callies R 1978 Thermometrische Untersuchungen bei unterschiedlichen Ultraschallintensitäten *Z. Physiother.* **30** 235–340

[41] Rathkolb O and Ammer K 1996 Skin temperature of the fingers after different methods of heating using a wax bath *Thermol. Österreich* **6** 125–9

[42] Ammer K and Schartelmüller T 1993 Hauttemperatur nach der Anwendung von Wärmepackungen und nach Infrarot-A-Bestrahlung *Thermol. Österreich* **3** 51–7

[43] Goodman P H, Foote J E and Smith R P 1991 Detection of intentionally produced thermal artifacts by repeated thermographic imaging *Thermology* **3** 253–60

[44] Dachs E, Schartelmüller T and Ammer K 1991 Temperatur zur Kryotherapie und Veränderungen der Hauttemperatur am Kniegelenk nach Kaltluftbehandlung *Thermol. Österreich* **1** 9–14

[45] Rathkolb O, Schartelmüller T, Hein L and Ammer K 1991 Hauttemperatur der Lendenregion nach Anwendung von Kältepackungen unterschiedlicher Größe und Applikationsdauer *Thermol. Österreich* **1** 15–24

[46] Ammer K 1996 Occurence of hyperthermia after ice massage *Thermol. Österreich* **6** 17–20

[47] Danz J, Callies R and Hrdina A 1981 Einfluß einer abgestuften Vakuumsaugmassage auf die Hauttemperatur *Z. Physiother.* **33** 85–92

[48] Eisenschenk A and Stoboy H 1985 Thermographische Kontrolle physikalisch-therapeutischer Methoden *Krankengymnastik* **37** 294

[49] Kainz A 1993 Quantitative Überprüfung der Massagewirkung mit Hilfe der IR-Thermographie *Thermol. Österreich* **3** 79–83

[50] Rusch D and Kisselbach G 1984 Comparative thermographic assessment of lower leg baths in medicinal mineral waters (Nauheim Springs) *Recent Advances in Medical Thermology* ed E F J Ring and B Phillips (New York: Plenum) pp 535–40

[51] Ring E F J, Barker J R and Harrison R A 1989 Thermal effects of pool therapy on the lower limbs *Thermology* **3** 127–31

[52] Ammer K 1994 Einfluß von Badezusätzen auf die Wärmeabstrahlung der Haut *ThermoMed* **10** 71–9

[53] Konermann H and Koob E 1975 Infrarotthermographische Kontrolle der Effektivität krankengymnastischer Behandlungsmaßnahmen *Krankengymnastik* **27** 397–400

[54] Smith B L, Bandler M K and Goodman P H 1986 Dominant forearm hyperthermia: a study of fifteen athletes *Thermology* **2** 25–8

[55] Melnizky P, Ammer K and Schartelmüller T 1995 Thermographische Überprüfung der Heilgymnastik bei Patienten mit Peroneusparese *Thermol. Österreich* **5** 97–102

[56] Ammer K 1995 Low muscular activity of the lower leg in patients with a painful ankle *Thermol. Österreich* **5** 103–7

[57] Mabuchi K, Chinzei T, Ikeda M, Saiti I and Fujimasa I 1995 Development of a data processing system for a high-speed thermographic camera and its use in analyses of dynamic

thermal phenomena of the living body *The Thermal Image in Medicine and Biology* ed K Ammer and E F J Ring (Vienna: Uhlen) pp 56–63
[58] Ring E F, Porto L O and Bacon P A 1981 Quantitative thermal imaging to assess inositol nicotinate treatment for Raynaud's syndrome *J. Int. Med. Res.* **9** 393–400
[59] Lecerof H, Bornmyr S, Lilja B, De Pedis G and Hulthen U L 1990 Acute effects of doxazosin and atenolol on smoking-induced peripheral vasoconstriction in hypertensive habitual smokers *J. Hypertens. Suppl.* **8** S29–33
[60] Tham T C, Silke B and Taylor S H 1990 Comparison of central and peripheral haemodynamic effects of dilevalol and atenolol in essential hypertension *J. Human Hypertension* **4** 77–83
[61] Natsuda H, Shibui Y, Yuhara T, Akama T, Suzuki H, Yamane K and Kashiwagi H 1994 Nitroglycerin tape for Raynaud's phenomenon of rheumatic disease patients—an evaluation of skin temperature by thermography *Ryumachi* **34** 849–53
[62] Ring E F J 1976 Computerized thermography for osteo-articular diseases *Acta Thermographica* **1** 166–73
[63] Roberts D L and Goodman P H 1987 Dynamic thermoregulation of back and upper extremity by computer-aided infrared imaging *Thermology* **2** 573–7
[64] Mabuchi K, Genno H, Matsumoto K, Chinzei T and Fujimasa I 1995 Autonomic thermoregulation and skin temperature: the role of deep body temperature in the determination of skin temperature *The Thermal Image in Medicine and Biology* ed K Ammer K and E F J Ring (Vienna: Uhlen) pp 121–9
[65] Damm F, Döring G and Hildebrandt G 1974 Untersuchungen über den Tagesgang von Hautdurchblutung und Haut-Temperatur unter besonderer Berücksichtigung der physikalischen Temperaturregulation *Z. Phys. Med. Rehabil.* **15** 1–5
[66] Heller M and Engel P 1982 Die Wirkung lokaler Wärmeanwendungen (Fango-Paraffin-Packungen) auf Kreislauf und Thermoregulation bei Applikation zu verschiedenen Tageszeiten *Z. Phys. Med. Baln. Med. Klim.* **11** 383–90
[67] Cena K 1984 Environmental heat loss *Recent Advances in Medical Thermology* ed E F J Ring and B Phillips (New York: Plenum) pp 81–93
[68] Engel J M 1983 *Kennzeichnung von Thermogrammen Thermologische Messmethodik* ed J-M Engel, U Flesch and F Stüttgen (Baden-Baden: Notamed) pp 176–81
[69] Schartelmüller T and Ammer K 1995 Räumliche Auflösung von Infrarotkameras *Thermol. Österreich* **5** 28–31
[70] Ring E F J and Dicks J M 1999 Spatial resolution of new thermal imaging systems *Thermol. Int.* **9** 7–14
[71] Ring E F J 1980 A thermographic index for the assessment of ischemia *Acta Thermographica* **5** 35–8
[72] Ring E F J 1980 Objective measurement of arthritis by thermography *Acta Thermographica* **5** 14–8
[73] Engel J-M and Saier U 1984 *Thermographische Standarduntersuchungen in der Rheumatologie und Richtlinien zu Deren Befundung* (München: Luitpold)
[74] Schartelmüller T and Ammer K 1996 Infrared thermography for the diagnosis of thoracic outlet syndrome *Thermol. Österreich* **6** 130–34
[75] Goodman P H, Murphy M G, Siltanen G L, Kelley M P and Rucker L 1986 Normal temperature asymmetry of the back and extremities by computer-assisted infrared imaging *Thermology* **1** 195–202

Chapter 2

The reproducibility of standard positions used for image capturing within the standard protocol for thermal imaging

We have established a protocol for capturing a series of images that covers the whole body of a healthy subject. The protocol defines a healthy subject as someone who has had no problems with mobility, no difficulty in caring for himself, no restrictions in performing normal activities, experienced no pain or discomfort and was not suffering from anxiety or depression. A total of 24 views of the body were specified and within these views, a total of 87 regions of interest (ROIs) were defined. The consistency of the standard views 'face', 'anterior left arm' and 'dorsal hands' has been evaluated. The distance, measured in pixels, from the upper or the lower edge of the image to anatomical landmarks was used for evaluation. The cross section tool of CTHERM was used for the determination of distances.

Positioning for the face varied in a very narrow way. However, any tilting of the head, which may be an important source in defining reference values, was not assessed in this procedure, but can easily performed by flipping the ROI (half of the face) of one side to the contralateral (figure 2.1).

Hand views varied in a wider range than the positioning of the face. This might be caused by a higher variability of hands between subjects. A different degree in spreading fingers may also contribute to this variation, as the definition of positioning 'middle fingers are parallel, thumbs do not touch' was not always followed.

With regard to the difficulty of positioning the arm, where three landmarks must be placed within the image, repeatability of this view was slightly better than the positioning of hands. Bending of the elbow at 90° was not always performed and this may have contributed to the variation of temperature readings (figure 2.2).

doi:10.1088/978-0-7503-1143-4ch2

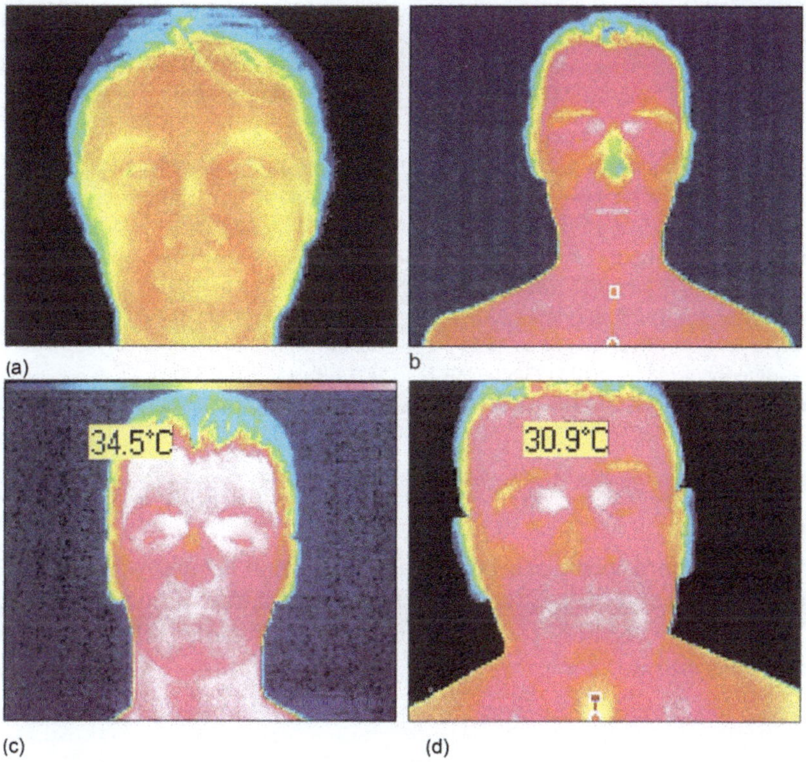

Figure 2.1. Human head in correct and incorrect views: (a) too close, (b) too far, (c) correct and (d) tilted to side not centered.

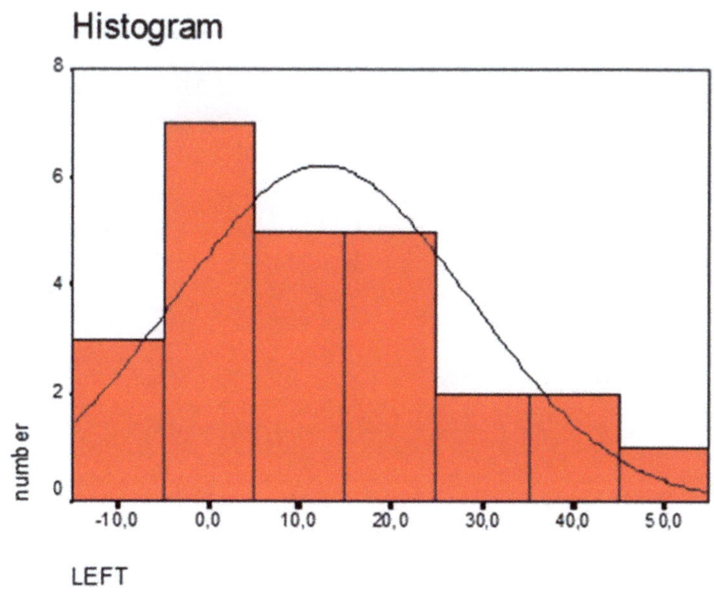

Figure 2.2. Reproducibility of the view for the left arm (anterior view). Distance to the left edge of the image (the outline of the deltoid muscle is within the image): 12.5 ± 16.0 pixels (5.9–19.1 pixels).

Table 2.1. Variation of the positions of all the investigated views (from Ammer K 2008 *Thermol. Int.* **18** 125–44).

View	Upper edge (pixels) mean ± SD (95% CI)	Lower edge (pixels) mean ± SD (95% CI)	Left side edge (pixels) mean ± SD (95% CI)
Face	0.5 ± 5.3 (−1.9)	4.0 ± 10.9 (−03 to 8.2)	
Dorsal neck	−8.4 ± 36.4 (−18.3 to 1.6)	122.6 ± 146.6 (82.6 to 162.6)	
Upper back	4.5 ± 9.9 (0.8 to 8.2)	28.1 ± 22.0 (19.9 to 36.4)	
Anterior left arm	22.4 ± 33.0 (8.7 to 36.0)	15.8 ± 15.4 (9.5 to 22.2)	12.5 ± 16.0 (5.9 to 19.1)
Dorsal hands	41.8 ± 17.8 (35.5 to 48.2)	33.2 ± 22.3 (25.3 to 41.5)	
Both knees anterior	80.7 ± 47.3 (60.7 to 100.7)	84.3 ± 37.0 (68.6 to 99.9)	
Lateral right leg	16.7 ± 21.0 (5.9 to 27.5)	17.2 ± 15.8 (9.0 to 25.3)	
Lower back	17.1 ± 4.2 (8.6 to 25.6)	16.3 ± 4.6 (16.3 ro 34.9)	
Both ankles anterior	158.8 ± 12.2 (133.6 to 184.1)	54.9 ± 9.1 (36.1 to 37.8)	
Plantar feet	31.0 ± 24.1 (23.2 to 38.7)	25.7 ± 23.1 (18.3 to 33.1)	

The repeatability of standard views varies by the body regions investigated (table 2.1).

However, standard views can be reproduced within a narrow range by different investigators. Reference values for the surface temperature of body regions based on images captured according to our protocol will mainly reflect the individual temperature variation.

IOP Publishing

Infrared Imaging
A casebook in clinical medicine
Kurt Ammer

Chapter 3

The reliability of temperature readings from selected standard views for thermal imaging

The definition of regions of interest (ROIs) for temperature measurements must meet two challenges. First, the region must capture as much information as possible from the body area of interest and second, the positioning of the region must show a high degree of reproducibility. Together with the use of standard views, reproducible temperature readings from ROIs will reduce the variability of temperature to individual features of the subjects investigated.

The inter-operator reliability of temperature measurements of three ROIs on the view 'anterior arm' was evaluated for five newly trained investigators (figure 3.1).

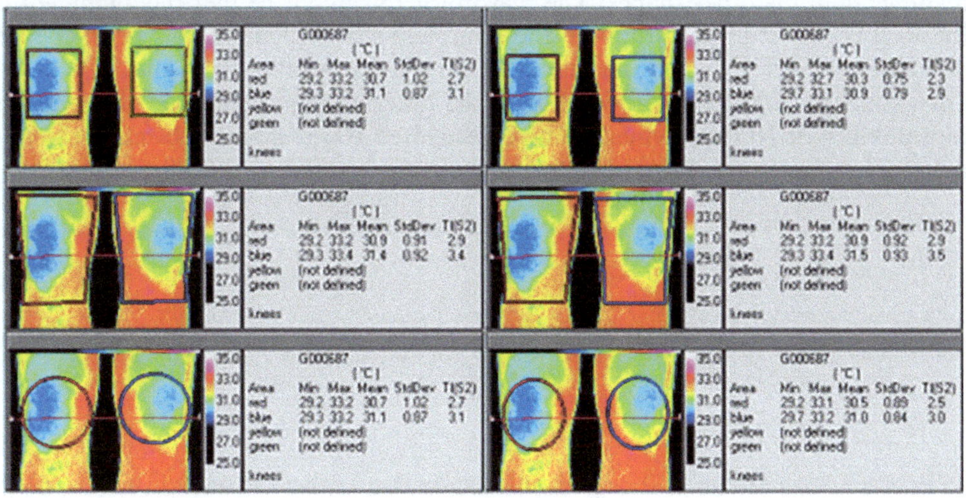

Figure 3.1. Reproducibility of read-outs of ROIs on thermal images of knees.

doi:10.1088/978-0-7503-1143-4ch3

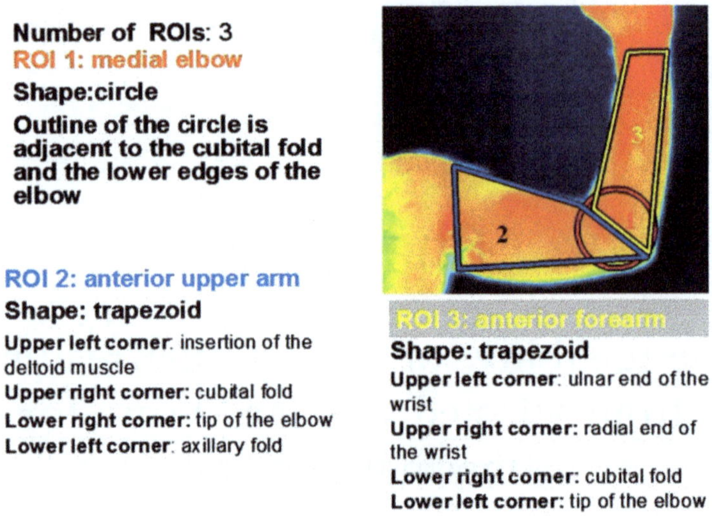

Figure 3.2. Examples of the ROIs for analysis.

In this experiment one thermal image of the anterior arm was given to the five individuals, who evaluated the thermal image twice following the protocol on standard views and the definition of the ROIs. This evaluation resulted in deviations from the mean temperature of the ROIs of between 0.001 °C and 0.10 °C at the elbow, between 0.06 °C and 0.27 °C at the upper arm and between 0.02 °C and 0.1 °C at the lower arm. The mean difference between the first and second measurements of individual investigators was 0.024.

In another experiment, a circle, a square and an hourglass shaped area were applied to the same image in the standard view 'anterior knee' by three newly trained investigators. Using the hourglass shape revealed a better precision of temperature readings than the other shapes. The reason for this might be that the alignment of the ROI is easiest to perform with the hourglass shape (figure 3.2). The inter-rater reliability coefficient α and the interclass correlation coefficient of the ROI 'lower arm', and the hourglass shaped ROI at the anterior knee confirmed the excellent repeatability of ROI placement. The investigated ROIs show high reliability and therefore the reference values created in such way are highly credible.

Chapter 4

The influence of colour scale on the accuracy of infrared thermal images*

A common definition of an infrared thermal image is 'a map of temperature distribution on the surface of the object image'. Consequently, thermal images are often regarded as two-dimensional temperature measurements and evaluations of the accuracy of thermal images are mostly restricted to the accuracy and reproducibility of temperature measurements, where accuracy is the 'closeness of agreement between a measured quantity value and a true value of a measureand'. The smaller the measurement error the better the accuracy. Although accuracy is sometimes understood as the closeness of agreement between measured quantity values that are being attributed to the measurand, the term 'accuracy' must not be used synonymously with the term 'measurement trueness', which is defined as 'closeness of agreement between the average of an infinite number of replicate measured quantity values and a reference quantity value' [1]. The common limits of measurement errors of infrared thermal imaging devices are ±2 °C [2].

Repeatability is defined as repeating a defined measurement applying identical equipment, conditions and procedures, while reproducibility is the attempt to achieve the same measurement results using different equipment and/or conditions and/or procedures.

Whenever a thermal image is understood as a map of temperature values, accuracy will always be based on the closeness of agreement between the measured temperature and the true value of the temperature. The colour palette, irrespective of its composition, will not have any influence on the accuracy of the temperature readings as long as the temperature map is the primary output of the recording device of infrared radiation. In the case where a copy of a recorded infrared image is used for calibration of the software that evaluates the temperature distribution

*First published in Ammer K 2014 *Thermol. Int.* **24** 141–6.

within the image, differences in grey shades and colours compared to the original recorded image will affect the accuracy of the temperature readings.

The human eye is the organ that provides vision and images. A single eye generates a two-dimensional representation of any two- or three-dimensional object which reflects or emits light. Possessing two eyes allows us to see three-dimensional space and the high level image processing of the central nervous system perfectly overcomes the rather crude optical system of the eye by transforming poor quality optical images into sharp, colourful and three-dimensional vision.

An accurate image could be defined by the closeness of agreement between the image and the object imaged. Several physical measures are available [3] to quantify image quality and define in this way the accuracy of an image. Colour, tone (contrast), resolution (detail), sharpness (edges) and noise all contribute to image quality. In contrast to temperature measurements, image processing procedures, such as different colour palettes, isotherms and compression or extension of the temperature window, will affect the accuracy of the thermal image.

As we cannot see infrared rays with our visual organs, we can only compare the image generated from the infrared emittance of objects with the optical image produced by our eyes or other optical systems. The poor resolution of early thermal imagers compared to photographs (figure 4.1) has been mentioned repeatedly [4, 5]. The resolution of infrared for imaging is better the closer the wavelength of the infrared is to visible light. However, recent developments in infrared detector design and image processing has resulted in a high resolution of details in grey shade thermal images recorded in the infrared long wave domain (figure 4.2).The rainbow palette is the preferred colour scale for thermal images in medicine and biology [7]. Variations of the colour palette, especially for use in breast thermography, have been proposed

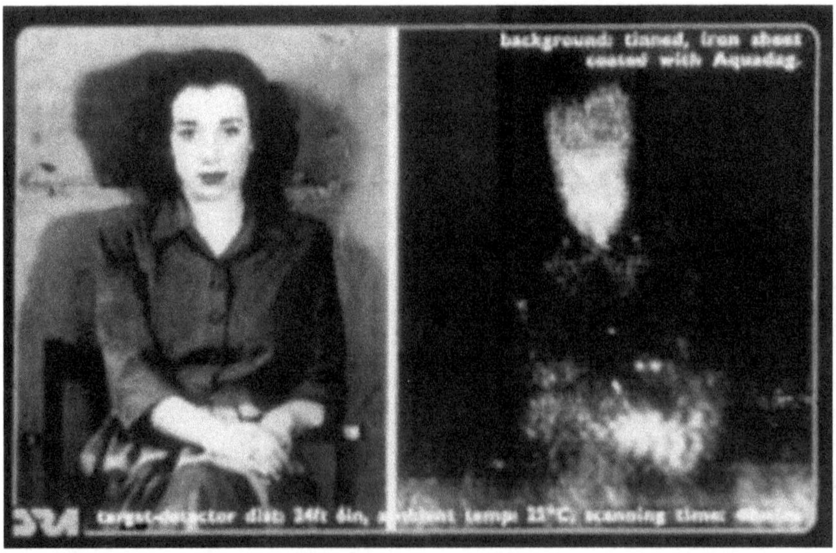

Figure 4.1. A comparison of photographic and thermal images in 1948 [4].

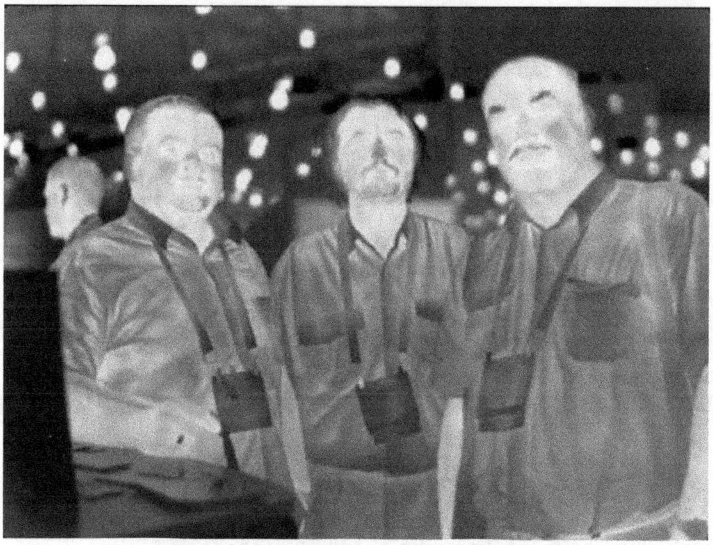

Figure 4.2. High definition infrared image recorded with a modern detector [6].

and evaluated [8, 9]. Vardasca suggested a rainbow based colour scale which had the highest acceptance among health professionals who were regularly involved in medical thermography [10]. However, none of these papers addressed the closeness of the thermal image to the visual image, although Zahedi *et al* [8] were aware that the pseudo-colouring of grey shade thermograms must not add information to the image and that a specific colour is not assigned to a specific temperature.

As chromatic colours resemble grey shades, false colour palettes add grey levels to the original grey shade image. Isotherms, which are commonly used in ten step increments in false coloured thermal images, add bands of additional grey shades and linear elements on the edges of each isotherm band due to the contrast of chromatic colours.

A series of processed thermal images of a patient with suspected CRPS (figure 4.3) show the effects of the different colour scales available in the FLIR software Thermocam Researcher Pro 2.1.

First, the image is displayed in continuous grey shades and ten grey shade isotherms, followed by continuous and ten isotherm iron palettes, continuous rainbow and ten isotherm rainbow colour scales and finally the ten isotherms medical scale (figure 4.4). It becomes obvious that the grey shade image is closest to the visual image, although the temperature distribution enhances the anatomy only in part and acts as a factor of deformation, which becomes more visible in the isotherm images. There, new areas are generated that do not correlate with any anatomical structure.

Compression of the temperature windows to widths of 9.1 °C and 6.4 °C slightly increases the resolution of the continuous grey shade images, but generates new areas and line elements in the grey isotherm image (figure 4.5). Narrowing the temperature window in false coloured isotherm thermograms induced a change in colours and also induced new shapes of areas not related to anatomy, leading in this way to a distortion of the visual image (figure 4.6).

N. I, female, age: 73 yrs.

After acclimatisation to a room temperature of 21 °C for 15 min with bare forearms, static thermal images of both hands were recorded and the following temperatures were obtained.

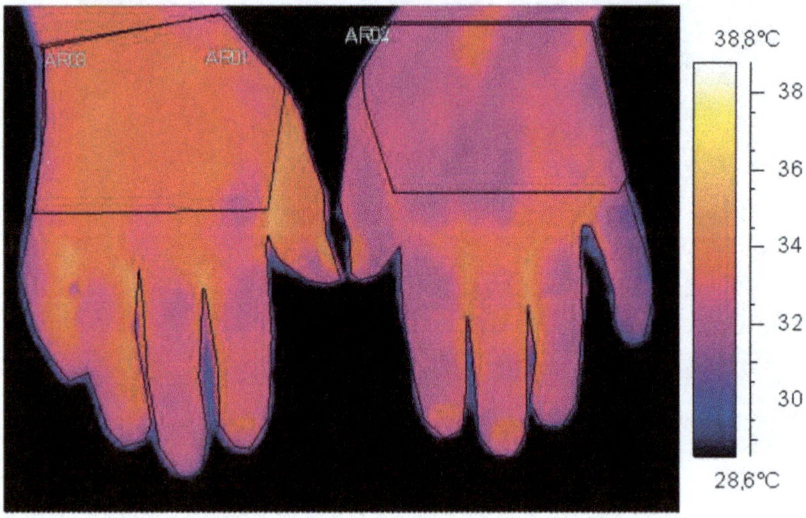

The right hand appears to be warmer than the left hand, the temperature difference of the total hand (AR01–AR02) is 0.75 °C, of the dorsal hand (AR03–AR04) it is 1.02 °C.

Measurement area	Temperature (°C)	Standard deviation
AR01 right hand, total	33.3	0.7
AR02 left hand, total	32.5	0.8
AR03 right hand, dorsal	33.5	0.4
AR04 left hand, dorsal	32.5	0.5
fo01	{ar1.avg}–{ar2.avg}	0.75
fo02	{ar3.avg}–{ar4.avg}	1.02

Figure 4.3. Original report for the patient with CRPS.

The brightness of an images is related to the grey levels of the image. One problem of colouring a grey shade thermal image arises from the fact that the grey level of a colour selected for enhancing a defined temperature band may differ from the grey level that already represents that temperature range in the original thermogram. In order to see these suspected changes, the thermograms displayed in the grey, iron, rainbow and medical palettes were imported into the software programme Adobe Photoshop CS5.1 (64 BIT) and all the images were transformed into grey shade images (figure 4.7) and histogram analysis was applied on these transformed grey images, shown in figure 4.8.

The histograms provide a detailed analysis of the visual impression that all methods of false colouring affect the grey levels of the original grey image. Separating the continuous colour into ten isothermal bands results in a change of the envelope of the grey level histograms. In the continuous scales, the distribution of grey levels occurs over a wide range with similar, but moderate frequencies. In the discontinuous scales, the

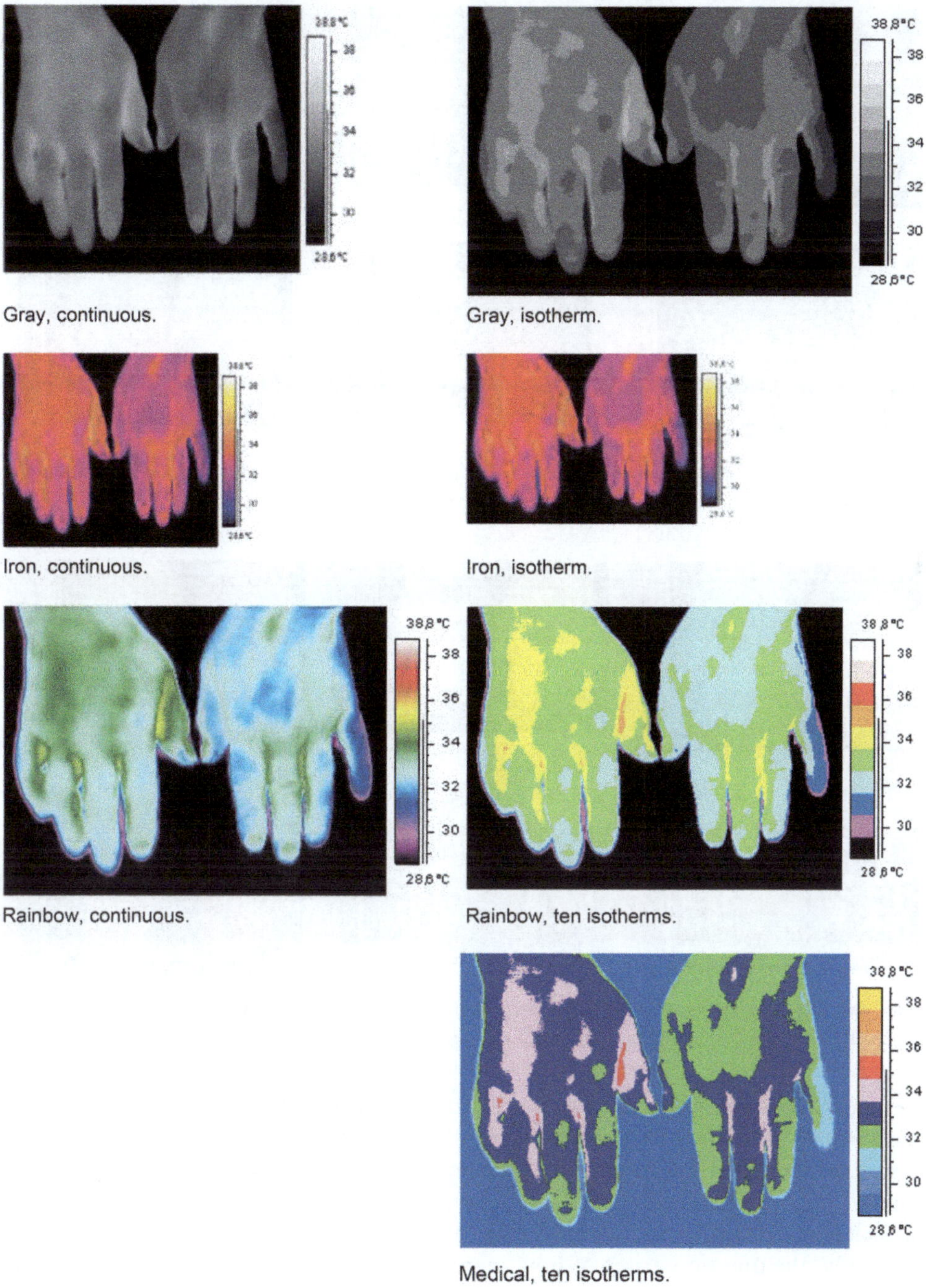

Figure 4.4. Images were recorded at a temperature window of 10 °C width.

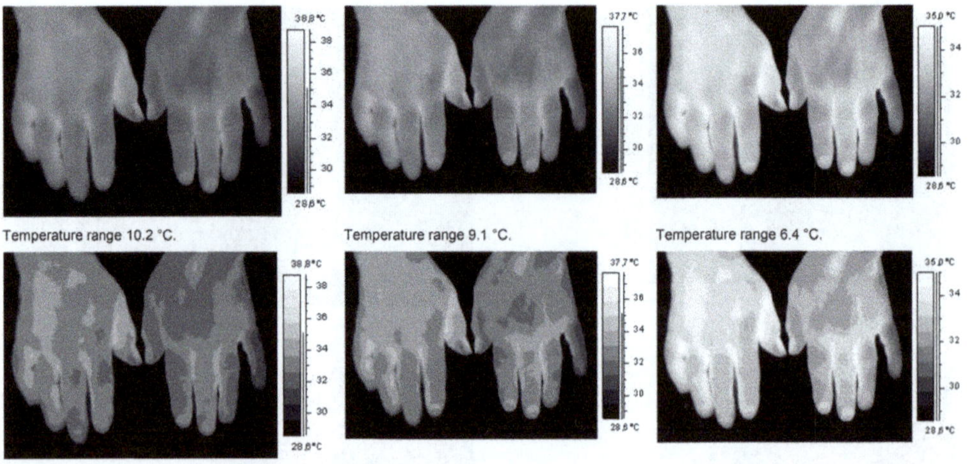

Figure 4.5. The effect of compression of the temperature window on the resolution of grey shade thermal images. Top row continuous grey shades, bottom row grey isotherms.

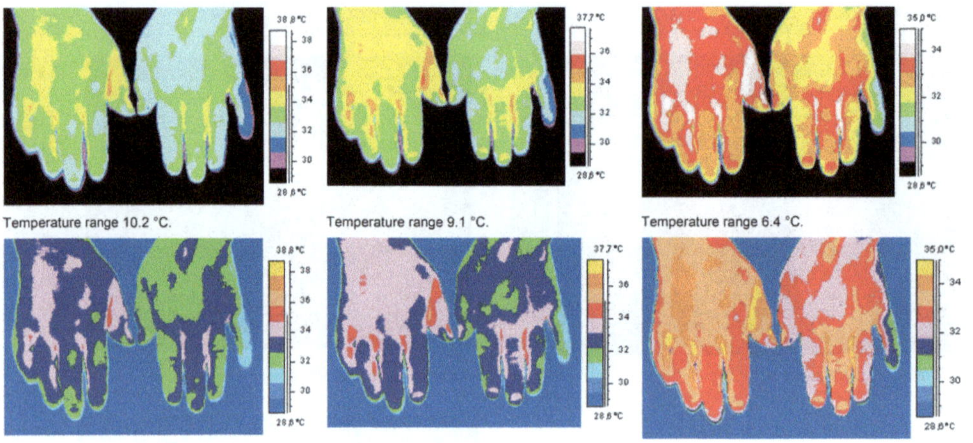

Figure 4.6. The effect of compression of the temperature window on the resolution in false coloured thermal images. Top row rainbow isotherms, bottom row medical isotherms.

average frequencies of the grey levels are much lower than in the continuous scales, but four peaks indicate maximum occurrence of these particular grey levels. The distribution of the grey levels of the continuous iron palette shows a better agreement with the original grey shade thermogram than the rainbow palette. All of the discontinuous scales have more similarities to each other than to the related continuous palettes.

Finally, the question arises of how many linear elements are added to the original thermogram by using different palettes. To this end, edge detection was performed in the grey versions of all the thermal images displayed with different palettes (figure 4.9). In order to equalize the grey level of the lines, automated level corrections were applied. This image processing resulted in images composed of grey linear elements and light grey areas. These images were also analysed by means of histograms (figure 4.10).

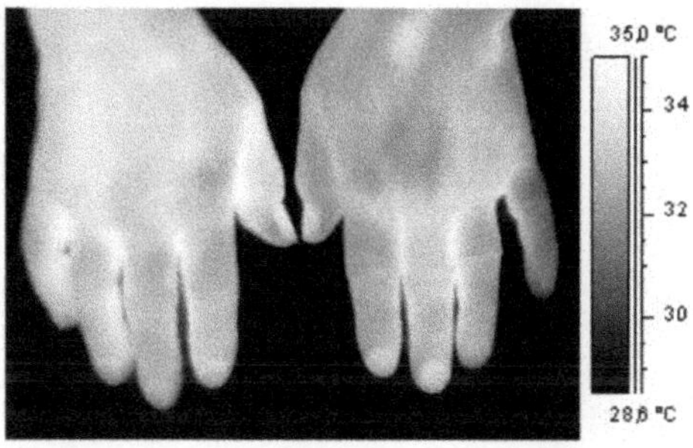

Grey, continuous.

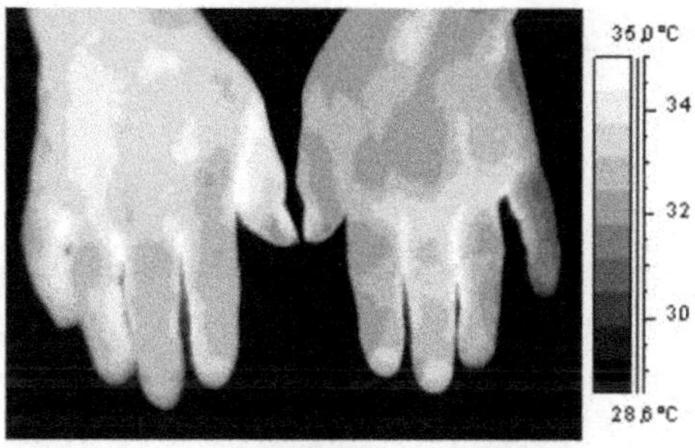

Grey, ten isotherms.

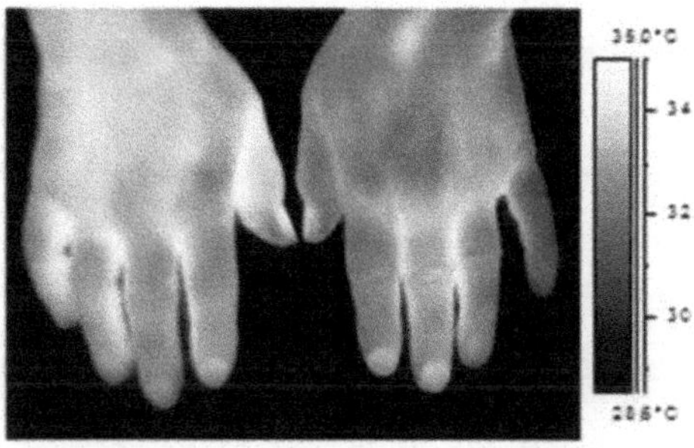

Iron, continuous.

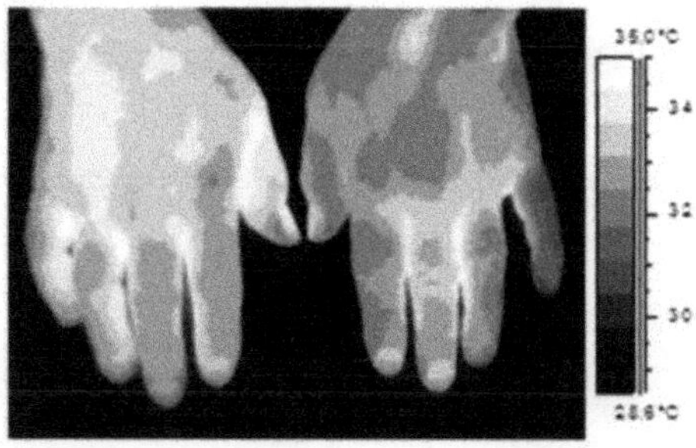

Iron, ten isotherms.

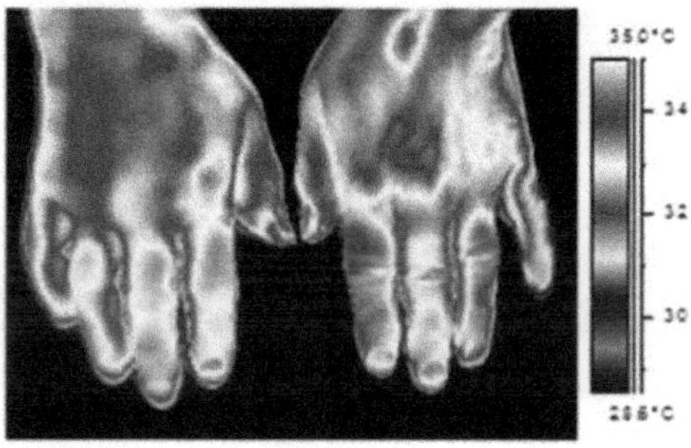

Rainbow, continuous.

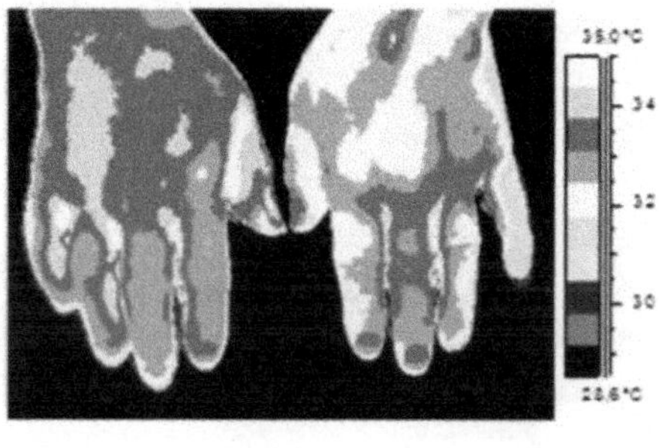

Rainbow, ten isotherms.

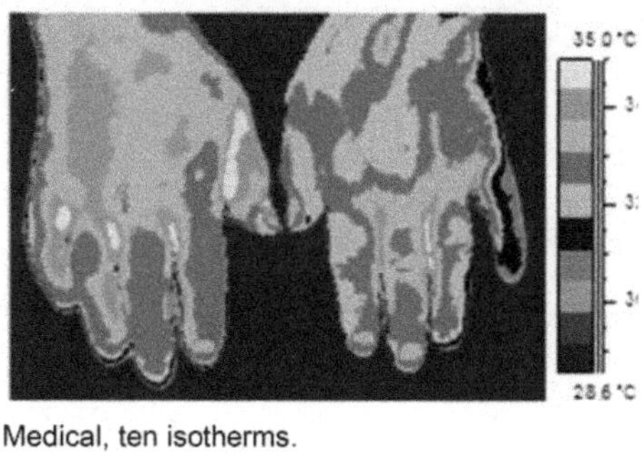

Medical, ten isotherms.

Figure 4.7. The temperature window was compressed to a width of 6.4 °C, the thermograms were transformed to grey shade images.

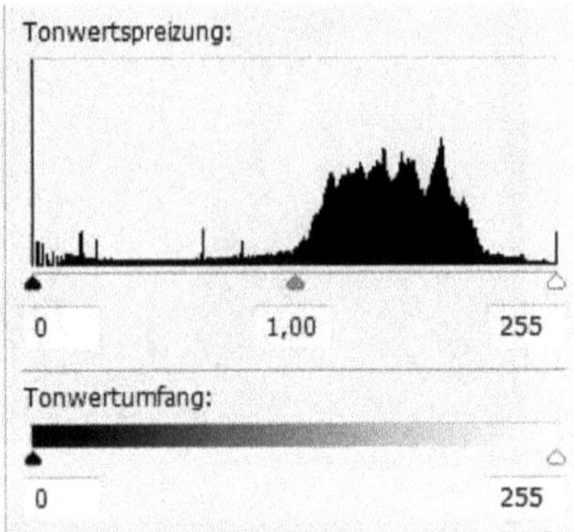

Grey, continuous.

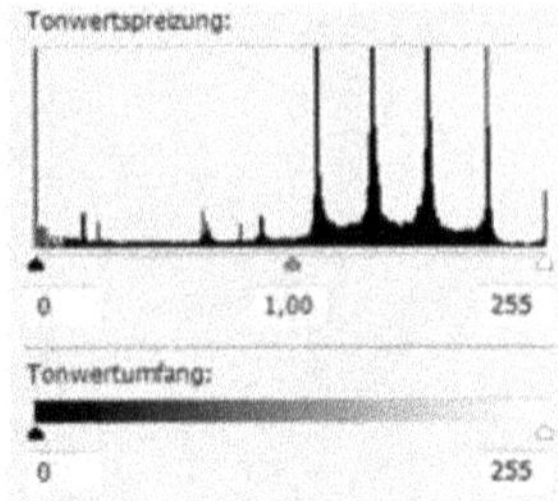

Grey, ten isotherms.

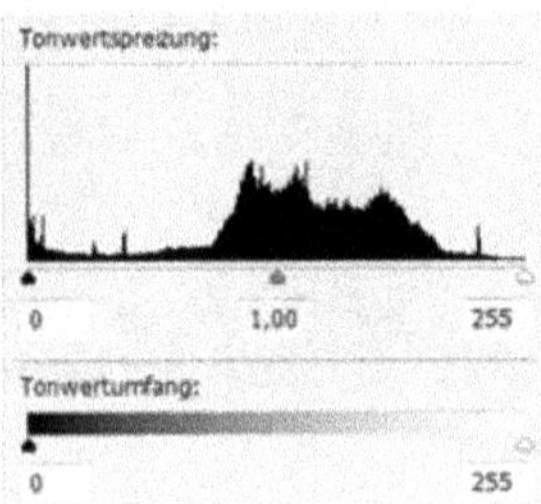

Iron, continuous.

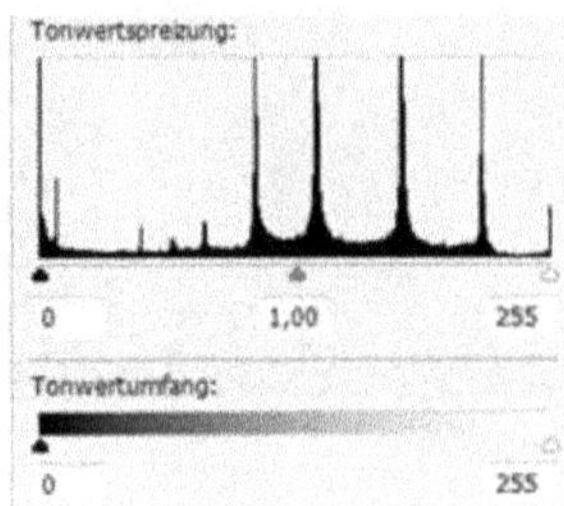

Iron, ten isotherms.

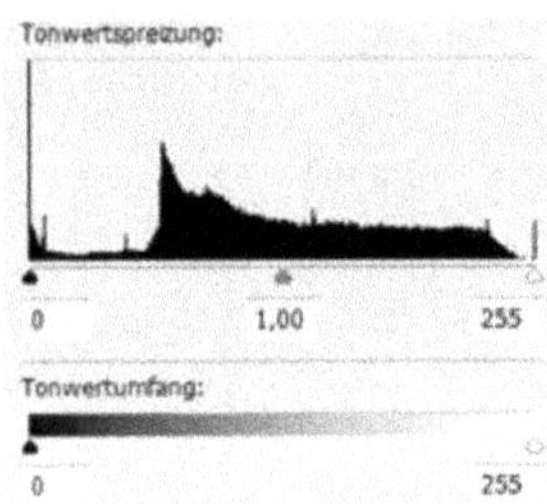

Rainbow, continuous.

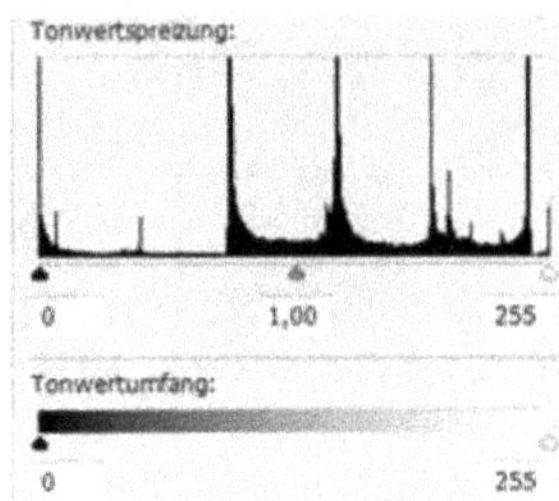

Rainbow, ten isotherms.

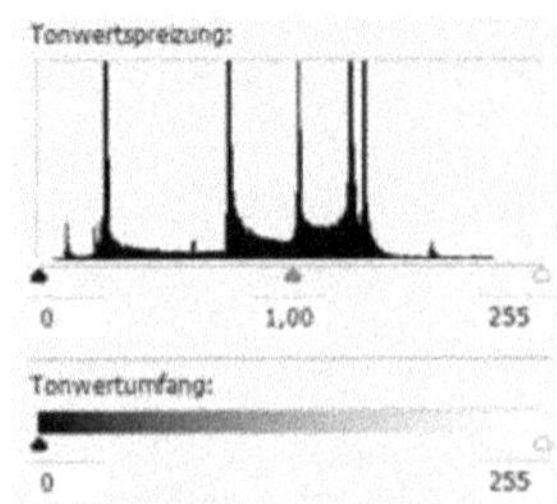

Medical, ten isotherms.

Figure 4.8. Grey level histograms of the thermal images shown in figure 4.7.

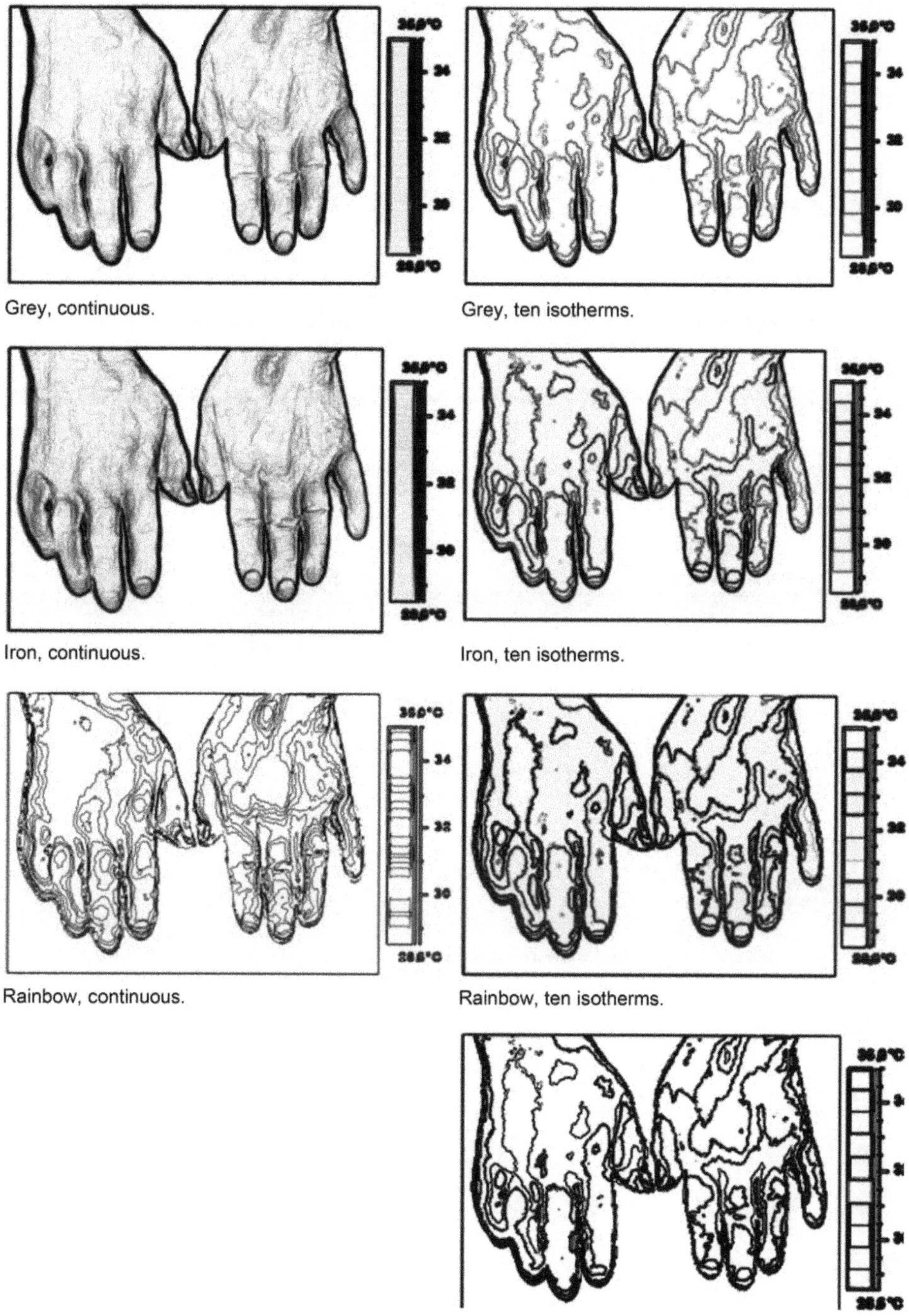

Figure 4.9. The temperature window was compressed to a width of 6.4 °C. The thermograms were transformed to grey shade images, automated level corrections was applied and edge detection was performed.

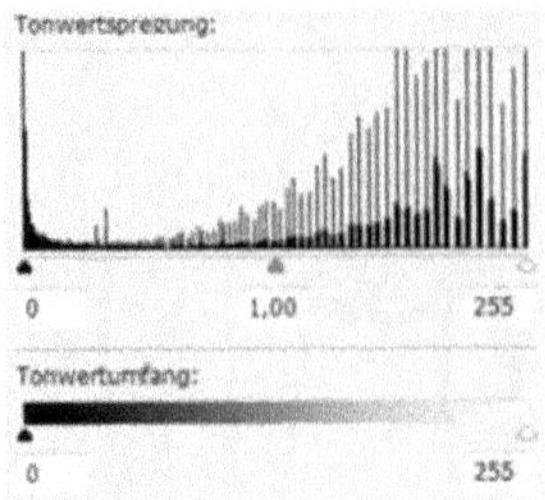

Grey, continuous.

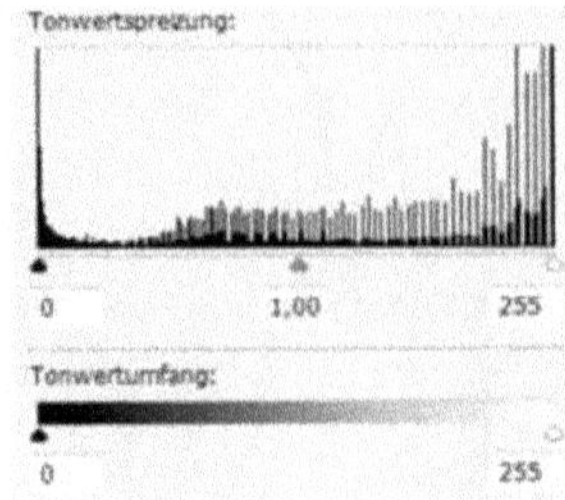

Grey, ten isotherms.

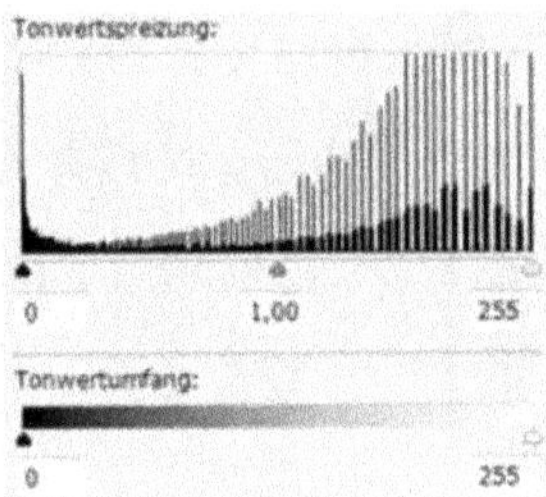

Iron, continuous.

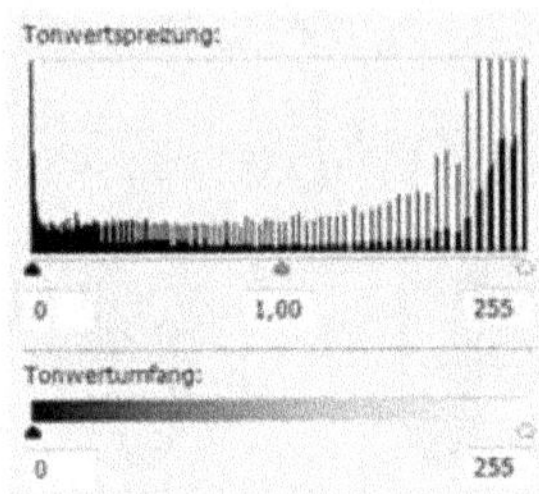

Iron, ten isotherms.

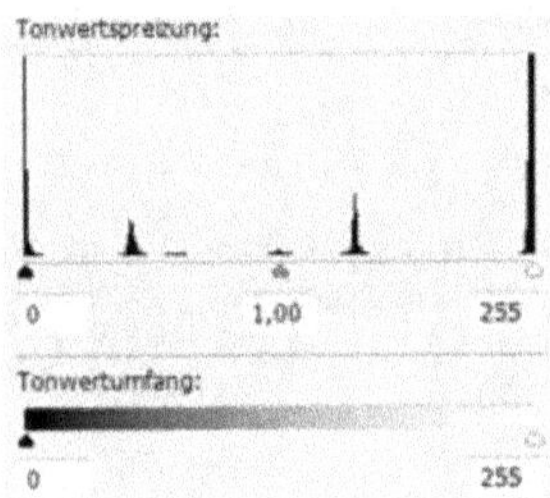

Rainbow, continuous.

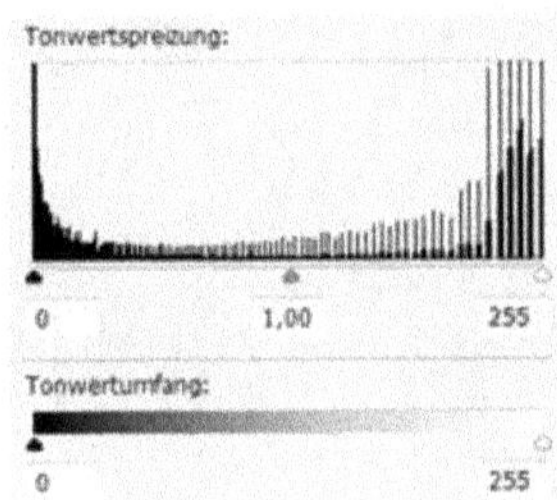

Rainbow, ten isotherms.

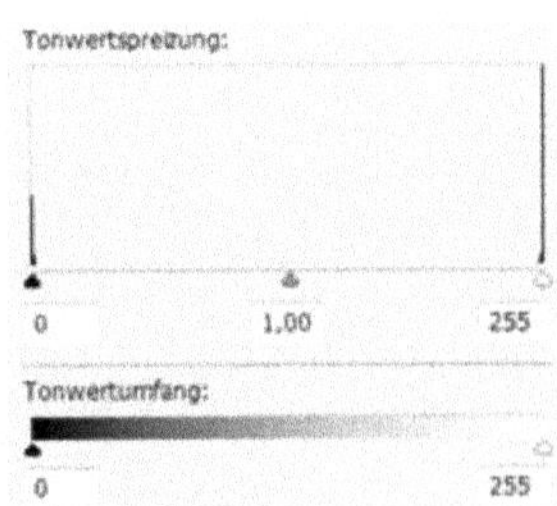

Medical, ten isotherms.

Figure 4.10. Grey level histograms of the thermal images shown in figure 4.9.

Surprisingly, the thus-processed continuous scale images look very much like pencil drawings of human hands, with many thin lines very close to each other. The isotherm images look like ink drawn landscape maps. The maximum grade of reduction was achieved in the medical palette showing only peaks at grey level 0 and grey level 255. The continuous rainbow palette was next in level of reduction. The continuous iron scale was very similar in grey level distribution to the original grey shade thermogram.

This series of processed and analysed thermograms clearly shows that false colouring affects resolution, grey levels and the likeness to the imaged object. In particular, the definition of isotherms, identifying a band of temperatures by a specific colour, adds a lot of distortion to the anatomy imaged. New areas and shapes are generated by isotherm images which are dependent on the temperature increment of the isotherm definition.

However, all of the thus-generated, so-called thermal signatures miss the most important finding in this patient: a difference in mean temperature >1 °C between both dorsal hands is strong support for the suspected diagnosis of CRPS. Hughen *et al* claimed that the asymmetry factor of temperature distribution has a greater diagnostic accuracy than mean temperature for the diagnosis of CRPS [11]. Conwell *et al* reported a paradoxical rewarming of the symptomatic CRPS limb when a cold stress was applied to a non-affected, asymptomatic extremity [12]. However, a typical thermal signature of CRPS has not yet been described and might not be detected, as the pathomechanism of CRPS affects more than one physiological system.

Finally, whenever the accuracy of thermal images is reported, the field of accuracy must be clearly stated, either using accurate temperature measurements, accurate imaging or the diagnostic accuracy of the technique.

References

[1] JCGM 2012 *VIM3: International Vocabulary of Metrology: Basic and General Concepts and Associated Terms* 3rd edn (BIPM: Paris) 200:2012

[2] Plassmann P, Ring E F J and Jones C D 2006 quality assurance of thermal imaging systems in medicine *Thermol. Int.* **16** 10–15

[3] Jacobson R 1995 Image quality criteria for hard copy from electronic images *The Thermal Image in Medicine and Biology* ed K Ammer and E F J Ring (Vienna: Uhlen) pp 111–20

[4] Cuthbertson G 1995 Development of IR detection in the UK *The Thermal Image in Medicine and Biology* ed K Ammer and E F J Ring (Vienna: Uhlen) pp 21–32

[5] Ring E F J 2003 The historical development of thermometry and thermal imaging in medicine *Thermol. Int.* **13** 53–57

[6] Ring E F J 2009 TTP 2009 Conference report *Thermol. Int.* **19** 128–9

[7] Ring E F J and Ammer K 2000 The technique of infrared imaging in medicine *Thermol. Int.* **10** 7–14

[8] Zahedi Z, Sadri S, Soltani M and Tehrani M K 2011 Breast disease detection and pseudo-coloring presentation for gray infrared breast images *IEEE Communications and Photonics Conf. and Exhibition* pp 1–8

[9] Aghdam N S, Amin M M, Tavakol M E and Ng E Y K 2013 Designing and comparing different color map algorithms for pseudo-coloring breast thermograms *J. Med. Imaging Health Inform.* **3** 487–93

[10] Vardasca R and Gabriel J 2014 A proposal of a standard rainbow false color scale for thermal medical images *Quantitative Infrared Thermography Conf. (7–11 July 2014, Bordeaux)* paper 170

[11] Huygen F J, Niehof S, Klein J and Zijlstra F J 2004 Computer-assisted skin video-thermography is a highly sensitive quality tool in the diagnosis and monitoring of complex regional pain syndrome type I *Eur. J. Appl. Physiol.* **91** 516–24

[12] Conwell T D, Hobbins W B and Giordano J 2010 Sensitivity, specificity and predictive value of infrared cold water autonomic functional stress testing as compared with modified IASP criteria for CRPS *Thermol. Int.* **20** 60–68

IOP Publishing

Chapter 5

New standards for fever screening with thermal imaging systems*

5.1 Introduction

In recent years, pandemic influenza viral infections have triggered concerns about the ever increasing mobility of populations, especially in air travel. Limiting exposure to fellow travellers who may be suffering from a febrile high temperature has been employed with some success. Pandemic influenza is a virulent form that causes global outbreaks or pandemics of serious illness in humans. Because there is little natural immunity, the disease can easily spread from individual to individual. In 1918, 1958 and 1968, there were pandemic outbreaks in the United States with varying degrees of morbidity and virulence. Children under 18 years of age tended to have the highest rates of illness, though not of severe disease and death [1]. There was initial interest in the possibility of using infrared imaging to identify fever arising from the severe acute respiratory syndrome (SARS) outbreak in Southeast Asia in 2003. Ng *et al* [2] evaluated the data from 502 subjects in Singapore and showed that the technique held promise; the best and most practical site for measurement is in the eye region, where the maximum temperature is recorded.

Infrared thermal imaging has in recent years become more accessible and affordable as a means of remote sensing for human body temperature. Historically, a clinical fever was checked and diagnosed with a clinical thermometer, and these devices have been slowly replaced by infrared radiometers mainly for inner ear temperature measurement. However, the number of scientific reports and papers confirming the reliability of such infrared methods are limited. Furthermore, there is a need for a critical technique, which has not always been well defined in these publications [3]. Nevertheless, infrared imaging for fever screening has been in use since 2006 in international airports, most

*First published in Ring E F J, Jung A, Kalicki B, Żuber J, Rustecka A and Vardasca R 2013 *J. Mech. Med. Biol.* **13** 1350045.

of which do not involve an optimal technique. For this reason, the International Organization for Standardization (ISO) produced two documents in 2008 and 2009—ISO TC121/SC3-IEC SC62D and ISO/TR 13154:2009 ISO/TR 80600 [4, 5].

These new standards are applicable to the use of thermal imaging in fever screening locations such as airports, public places and entrances to hospitals. Until now, the threat of a pandemic infection has not been raised sufficiently high to require such sweeping measures. The need for airport screening however, became apparent after the outbreak of the highly contagious infection SARS in 2003–4. A number of thermal imaging systems were hastily employed in Southeast Asia, but were mainly used for crowd surveillance. It is now evident that this is not an efficient way to identify passengers with a raised temperature and, not surprisingly, only a small number of suspected cases of fever were discovered by this approach. The Singapore Standards authority published a guidance document which pointed the way to a more stringent approach to identifying passengers with a detectable increase in facial temperature. These documents were referred to the ISO for consideration. An international group of experts were brought together and after a series of meetings, the Singapore documents were extended and updated following ISO procedures. The final documents were published as the ISO TC 121/SC3-IEC SC62D (*Particular Requirements for the Basic Safety and Essential Performance of Screening Thermographs for Human Febrile Temperature Screening*) in 2008 [4]. This was followed by a technical report especially written for organizations purchasing and deploying thermal imaging cameras for screening—ISO/TR 13154:2009 ISO/TR 80600 (*Medical Electrical Equipment–Deployment, Implementation and Operational Guidelines for Identifying Febrile Humans Using a Screening Thermograph*) [5].

These documents essentially focus on the minimal requirements for a radiometric camera (i.e., capable of measurement) that is required to measure with the optimal certainty the small area at the inner corner of the human eye, with at least nine pixels. It was also shown that non-radiometric cameras that have been used in some locations are not designed for temperature measurement and should therefore not be used. The standard also requires the subject to be stationary and close to the camera without angular distortion to optimize the target site, ruling out the common practice of distant surveillance of a moving crowd of subjects. One important issue that is key to the correct technique for fever detection is the positioning of both the camera and subject. Typical screening installations make use of cameras mounted at an angle to survey passing groups of passengers. The best site for temperature measurement is the inner corner (or canthus) of the eye. This requires the camera to be mounted up close and level with the eyes, thus providing a cluster of image pixels in the region of interest (ROI).

The second document is a guide for the authority responsible for implementing the standard for screening. The need for quality assurance, regular calibration checks, training and documentation are all described. Furthermore, there is a description of the optimum type of camera that should be purchased for the application. There is an implied responsibility in the correct operation of thermal imaging for screening, since a passenger with raised temperature can be stopped from travelling and mistakes could be open to litigation. Thermal imaging is indicated as the first stage only and the suspected passenger will then be diverted to a nurse or clinician whose task is to medically check the passenger with clinical thermometry or radiometry and record any relevant history of infection or infection exposure. Only if this test yields confirmation of fever would prevention from travel be implemented. This also would be dependent on the local Public Health orders that have been put in place due to the pandemic situation. Should this procedure become routine under non-pandemic situations, there may well be a need for more effective legislation to avoid contentious hold ups in the airport. Currently, eye recognition software has already been installed in some airports for passport verification and it would be possible to extend this procedure to a simultaneous temperature check by infrared imaging.

5.1.1 Camera specification

A further ISO group is now in operation to develop a new document dealing with the descriptive specifications for infrared cameras. The need for this is driven by the variability across the market in specification terminology for such cameras, which makes the comparison or selection of a suitable instrument more difficult for the purchaser and user. At the centre of this document is a detailed vocabulary list with definitions that when finalized, will be accepted by the participating National Standards organizations around the world.

The new document specifically applies to thermal imaging devices (thermal imagers). It is limited to devices that operate in the infrared waveband and those that are based on focal plane array detectors. It identifies and defines the essential technical data (parameters) that should be given by manufacturers when describing the performance of thermal imagers. The objective of the document is to ensure that any supplied technical data be provided in a consistent and unambiguous manner, with the same terminology used throughout the industry. This will greatly facilitate the user/purchaser when comparing thermal imagers from different suppliers. A normative reference cited is the 2008 publication on metrology values [4].

The following section deals with a number of definitions, terms and abbreviations. These include measurement uncertainty, ambient temperature effects, short-term stability (repeatability), long-term stability (reproducibility), operating temperature range, storage temperature range, image uniformity, measuring distance, influence of air humidity, etc.

The document will in effect be the first attempt to create a specific internationally agreed vocabulary relating to the parameters needed to define the performance of an infrared camera. It will be important to manufacturers and commissioners of thermal imaging equipment, provided that the industry does follow the terminology set out in the document.

5.1.2 Is the standard being applied?

So far, there has not been a radical change in the use of infrared cameras used for fever screening since the publication of the standard in 2009. However, it may require a longer time for more widespread adherence to this standard. In almost all cases, such standards are not enforceable by law, but must be publicized for their value to be recognized as ‘best practice’.

It is clearly important that definitions of camera performance and especially those relating to or influencing temperature measurement are precisely defined, understood and capable of being compared between different instruments designed for the same purpose. At present, there is a lack of conformity across the developing industry for infrared imaging in the descriptive literature provided to their customers. It is hoped that this new initiative will address this problem, but this will only happen with the full cooperation of the manufacturers and marketing organizations promoting infrared imaging systems.

One other important issue is the need for clinical studies to evaluate the concept of temperature measurement from the face for fever detection. The early work of Carl R A Wunderlich in the 19th century is constantly used in the principles of fever detection based on temperature. However, technology has radically changed and even his mercury-based clinical thermometer is out of favour in many countries. Current opinion on the relative merits of tympanic membrane radiometry is variable and the quality of instrumentation is not the same across the world. The National Physical Laboratory in the United Kingdom has developed special standard reference temperature devices for the calibration of tympanic membrane thermometers, but how much is known of the drift over time of these now heavily used devices? Some other systems sold include those that estimate body core temperature with an unknown and unproven algorithm; this cannot possibly be a reliable tool for screening large numbers of subjects.

5.1.3 A clinical study for fever detection in children

To investigate the usefulness of the new standard for thermal imaging, we studied a group of children in a paediatric hospital setting.

5.2 Method

Cohorts of children at the Paediatric Clinic in Warsaw were checked for fever by three different methods. The routine department procedure was carried out by a nurse using a clinical thermometer under the armpit (axilla) left there for a full 5 min. The subjects then entered a room for thermal imaging maintained at 22 °C–23 °C where they were seated before the FLIR infrared camera SC640. The image of the face was set to occupy at least 75% of the image and regions around the inner canthi (i.c.) were measured for temperature. A second area of interest over the forehead was also recorded as some claims have been made that forehead temperature would be an adequate target for fever. Both inner ear measurements (tympanic membrane) with a clinical radiometer were then recorded and documented, with the child's demographic data.

5.3 Results

A total of 402 children (table 5.1) were examined between 2006 and 2011. The majority of children in attendance at the hospital were not febrile; they were compared with those known to have a clinically defined fever and examined prior to medication. Of this group, 350 (85%) were found to be free from fever and 52 (15%) cases of definite fever were recorded. There were 192 males and 210 females.

Table 5.1. Age distribution of subjects.

Age	Number
<3	50
3–6	128
7–12	136
13–16	82
>16	6

Table 5.2. Temperature data: non-fevered group.

Afebrile	Mean temperature (°C)	Standard deviation	Number
Eyes i.c.	36.48	0.49	354
Forehead	36.44	0.65	326
Axilla	36.34	0.59	347
Ear	36.12	0.71	178

Table 5.3. Temperature data: fevered group (49% male; 51% female).

Febrile	Mean temperature (°C)	Standard deviation	Number
Eyes i.c.	38.9	0.84	52
Forehead	34.7	0.86	52
Axilla	38.9	0.68	52
Ear	37.4	1.41	24

All subjects had infrared thermograms and axilla recordings; not all subjects were measured using the ear tympanic membrane thermometer, due to equipment failure.

5.3.1 Temperature data

The data were analysed for differences between males and females, and no statistical differences were found for sex dependency. Similarly, for age dependency no statistical differences were found. In the control subjects (non-febrile), left eye versus right eye data were compared and found to be not significant. As a result, both readings were combined and the mean temperature of both eyes was used for each subject. Conventionally, temperatures of 38 °C and above were considered to be a fever case in children over 5 years of age and adults, while 37.5 °C and above was considered to be a fever case in subjects less than 5 years old. In this study, we have categorized all temperatures over 37.6 °C as fever. In most cases, the temperatures were higher than 38 °C.

From these data, it was shown that in febrile children, the eye temperature measurements and the thermometric axilla temperatures are statistically closer than those measured from the forehead (thermographic) or ear (tympanic membrane radiometer). The eye and axilla measurements as tabulated in tables 5.2 and 5.3 also showed more internal consistency than the others (reliability coefficient α of 0.724).

Table 5.4. Non-fevered group.

Pair	*r*	*n*	*p*
Eyes i.c./axilla	0.507	354	0.0006
Forehead/axilla	0.432	326	0.000
Tympanic/axilla	0.420	178	0.014

Table 5.5. Fevered group.

Pair	*r*	*n*	*p*
Eyes i.c./axilla	0.587	52	0.000
Forehead/axilla	0.432	52	0.022
Tympanic/axilla	0.276	24	0.267

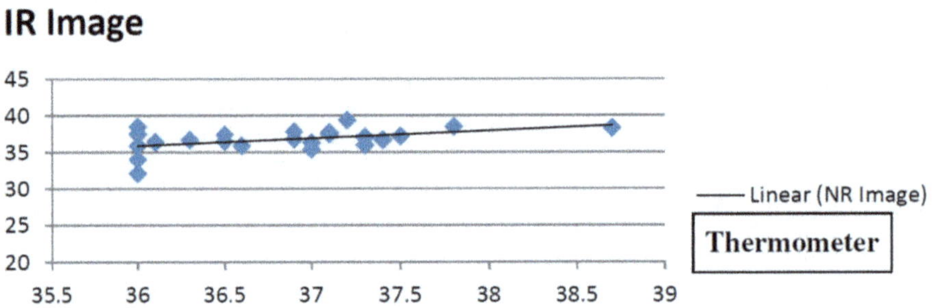

Figure 5.1. The relationship between the i.c. temperatures obtained using thermography and axilla temperatures measured using thermometry in a group of adults.

To examine the possible relationship between the different measurement sites and methods, Pearson correlation tests were performed on the temperature data. These data in tables 5.4 and 5.5 showed the existence of a linear relationship between the measurements between sites in the fever cases. This is highest when comparing the i.c. eye measurements from thermography and axilla temperatures measured using the clinical contact thermometer. The forehead temperatures and ear measurements correlated less well with statistical significance ($p < 0.1$).

A small group of adults (18 subjects measured on 24 occasions) were also assessed using axilla thermometry and infrared thermography (IRT) of the i.c. of the eyes. It was interesting to note that in two subjects with fever, lower temperatures were recorded by thermometry, probably due to profuse sweating at the site of measurement (male: 39.4 °C IRT and 37.2 °C axilla; female: 38.5 °C IRT and 36.0 °C axilla). All other readings (figure 5.1) showed a good relationship between the two sites and measurements.

5.4 Discussion

This study was performed on children in Warsaw, Poland according to the recommended technique described in the new ISO standards of 2008/9. The advantage of performing the study in a hospital environment was that the diagnosis was known prior to the study measurements, but was not conveyed to those undertaking the study until after the data had been examined. There were no cases of clinical fever that were undetected by the study. Treatment for fever was not commenced until after the assessments were made. Figure 5.2 shows two thermograms of the faces young male childen, on the left during fever and the right a normal healthy child of the same age. Figure 5.3 presents the inbuilt software for making spot temperature measurements over the eye, where the temperature difference from right to left is 0.2 °C. The ISO standard recommends a minimum of nine pixels to be measured at this anatomical site. Figure 5.4 illustrates the effect of thermal resolution on thermograms and the importance of using more pixels in the measurement areas.

To examine if another source of mild infection such as sinusitis could confound the data and cause a false positive result, six known cases of sinusitis were examined using the same protocol. In the case of sinusitis, there is often a bilateral increase in

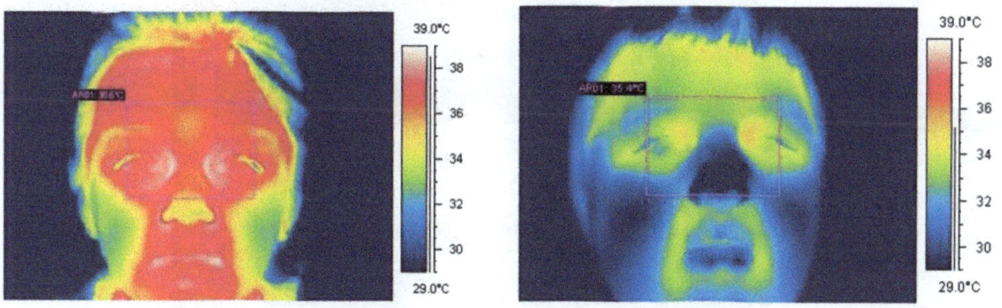

Figure 5.2. Thermograms of the faces of young male children. Left: during fever; right: a normal healthy child of the same age.

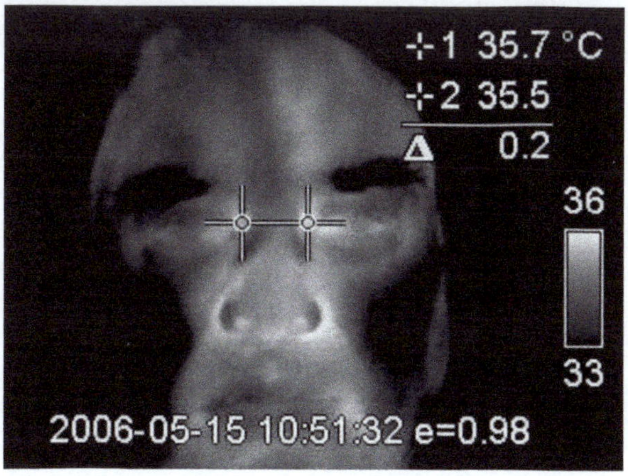

Figure 5.3. Inbuilt software for making spot temperature measurements over the eye, where the temperature difference between the right and left was 0.2 °C. However in repositioning, the two corresponding eye regions were of the same temperature. This illustrates the danger of using this system with very few pixels in the measuring area. The ISO standard recommends a minimum of nine pixels to be measured at this anatomical site.

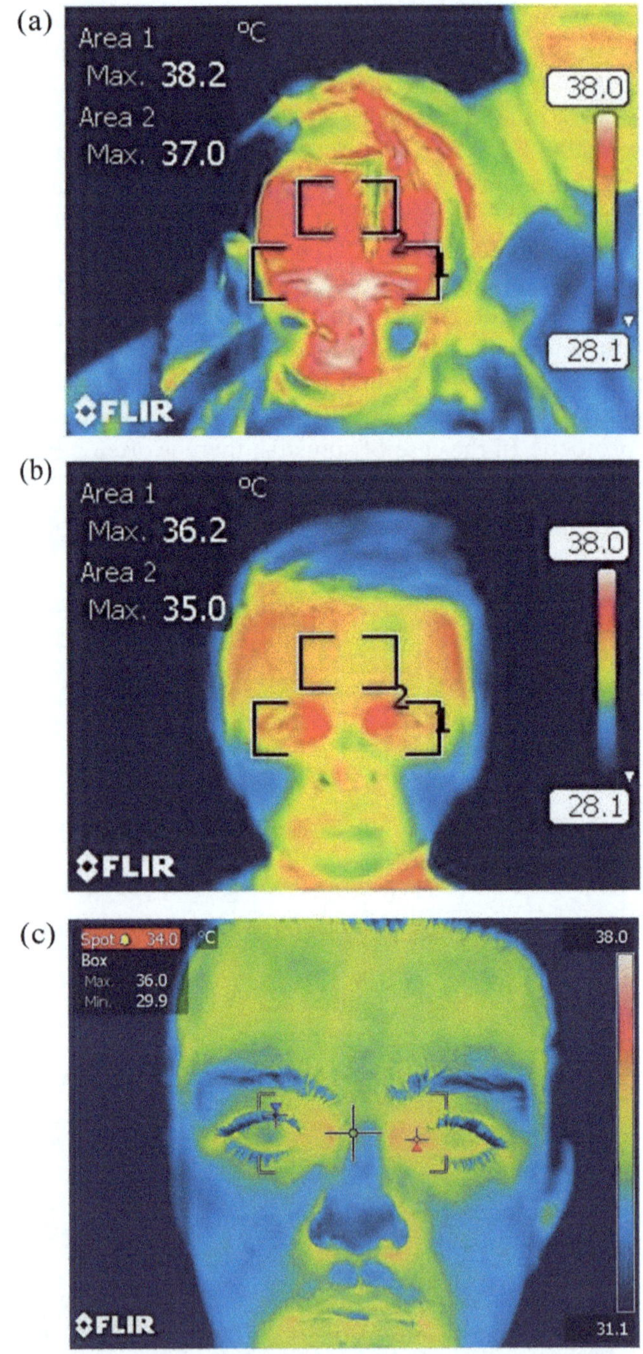

Figure 5.4. (*a*) Thermogram of a child with fever examined by a FLIR handheld i7 infrared camera. The resolution was lower, but the raised temperature is shown. However, here the maximum temperatures for the ROIs are shown and the accuracy will again depend on the number of pixels in the measurement. (*b*) Similar to (*a*) but for the face of a healthy child. (*c*) Thermogram of a higher resolution FLIR P640 camera with a better quality image and the possibility of using more pixels in the measurement areas.

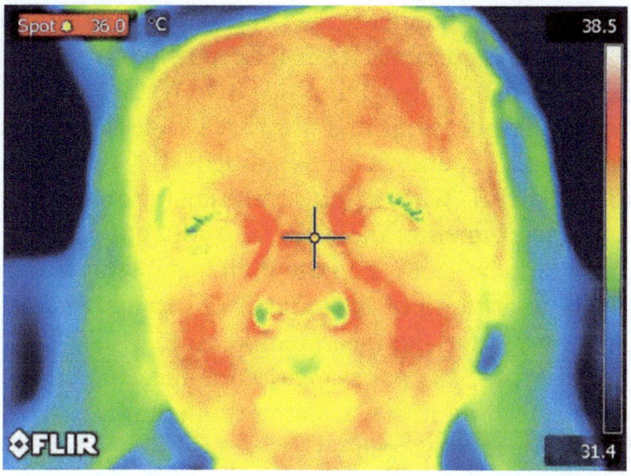

Figure 5.5. Thermogram of a six-year-old girl with sinusitis. There are clear differences in this condition from fever.

heat affecting the face, rarely causing an increase in the i.c. temperatures. The clinical fever cases in this study showed excellent symmetry, so a close correlation was always found between the left and the right eyes, in both febrile and afebrile patients. Those with sinusitis or dental infection showed a characteristic localized and asymmetric temperature increase. An example of sinusitis from our study was incorporated in the ISO document illustrating the differences from a fever case in a 10-year-old child as shown in figure 5.5.

The examination room used was thermally stable and air-conditioning could be operated prior to a clinical session if required. However, unlike the normal protocols recommended for clinical tests using infrared imaging, the patients were not required to rest and stabilize their body systems prior to the test. This would not be practical in a traveller screening situation and the concept of the i.c. of the eye being the most stable site for measurement was borne out by this study. The forehead on the other hand, also measured from the thermogram using a rectangular ROI occupying some 60% of the exposed area, did not show such consistency.

For the most efficient positioning of the subject before the camera, a stool was used, which limited the range of height adjustment required for the camera stand. This was a counterbalanced single pillar stand as used in photographic studios. The ISO document specifically warns of the potential for error in reproducible positions when using a pan and tilt head tripod for the infrared camera mount.

This study has also endorsed the methodology recommended in the ISO document for fever screening, where a close up stationary image is recorded of the subject's face. With the current infrared cameras, even using the best available system, the error could be as high as 0.4 °C, which is a large proportion of the actual difference in temperatures found between afebrile and febrile cases. It is therefore clear that a camera mounted more than 1 m away from the subject, and possibly also at an oblique angle, will fail to have sufficient pixels in the relatively small target area of the i.c. of an eye. Increasing the number of pixels over the measurement site is not only good, but essential practice in this application.

Fever screening in a global pandemic has yet to be taken seriously, but it is clear that there can be legal repercussions from false positive measurements due to bad technique or inadequate technology. False negative results in mass screening of this kind would have serious implications and must be avoided [6]. Suzuki *et al* [7] studied the effect of environment temperature in 50 adults. They compared the temperature of the face recorded by IRT with axilla thermometry (used to approximate core temperature) and tympanic membrane radiometry at both 16 °C and 20 °C. They found ear measurements to be more accurate than facial temperatures. However, they did not give a detailed description of the manner of thermal imaging data acquisition and implied that they only used the mean temperature of the face, not the i.c. of the eyes. From their conclusions, tympanic membrane measurements could be effective for body temperature screening in a warm environment only, which differs from the ISO recommendations for fever screening.

In this study, the commercial software proved entirely adequate for the analysis of two regions of the face. However, some recent studies have proposed software that will automatically track the human face and obtain measurements with minimal intervention by the operator. This approach will lead the way to rapid screening in the future [8–11].

5.5 Conclusion

The use of an infrared radiometric camera can be a reliable tool for the detection of fever in children. The technique recommended by the ISO in document TR 13154:2009 ISO/TR 80600 is endorsed by the results of this study. There was a significant difference between the temperatures measured in non-fevered patients and those with known fever, with the thermal imaging of the eye region being the most rapid non-contact site for measurement. As more studies are carried out in future, using the optimal criteria described, more objective data from both healthy and febrile subjects can be evaluated. At present, the poorly controlled use of thermal imaging for fever screening is most unlikely to prove to be an effective tool.

Acknowledgments

We are extremely grateful for the full cooperation FLIR Infrared Systems, Warsaw, the regular support of Mr Pawel Rutkowski and the loan of the infrared camera. We also thank the staff and patients of the Military Institute of Medicine, Warsaw for their willing participation in this study.

References

[1] US Department of Homeland Security 2006 *Pandemic Influenza: Preparedness, Response and Recovery. Guide for Critical Infrastructure and Key Resources* http://www.flu.gov/planning-preparedness/business/cikrpandemicinfluenzaguide.pdf 2006

[2] Ng E Y K, Kaw G J and Chang W M 2004 Analysis of IR thermal imager for mass blind fever screening *Microvasc. Res.* **68** 104–9

[3] Dodd S R, Lancaster G A, Craig J V, Smyth R L and Williamson P R 2006 In a systematic review, infrared ear thermometry for fever diagnosis in children finds poor sensitivity *J. Clin. Epidemiol.* **59** 354–7

[4] International Organization for Standardization (ISO) 2008 *Particular Requirements for the Basic Safety and Essential Performance of Screening Thermographs for Human Febrile Temperature Screening* TC121/SC3-IEC SC62D

[5] International Organization for Standardization (ISO) 2009 *Medical Electrical Equipment—Deployment, Implementation and Operational Guidelines for Identifying Febrile Humans Using a Screening Thermograph* ISO/TR 13154:2009 ISO/TR 8-600

[6] Ng E Y K 2005 Is thermal scanner losing its bite in mass screening of fever due to SARS? *Med. Phys.* **32** 93–7

[7] Suzuki T, Wada K, Kagitani H, Arioka T, Maeda K and Kida K 2010 The validity of mass body temperature screening with ear thermometers in a warm thermal environment, Tohoku *J. Exp. Med.* **222** 89–95

[8] Strakowska M, Strzelecki M and Wiecek B 2011 Automatic measurement of human body temperature in the eye canthi using a Thermovision camera *Thermol. Int.* **21** 57–8

[9] Bajwa U I, Taj I A and Bhatti Z E 2011 A comprehensive comparative performance analysis of Laplacian faces and Eigen faces for face recognition *Imaging Sci. J.* **59** 32–40

[10] Ng E Y K and Acharya U R 2009 A review of remote-sensing infrared thermography for indoor mass blind fever screening in containing an epidemic *IEEE Eng. Med. Biol.* **28** 76–83

[11] SPRING Singapore 2013 *Specification for Thermal Imagers for Human Temperature Screening—Implementation Guidelines.* Part 2 of Singapore Standards (Singapore: SPRING Singapore)

B Kalicki, A Jung, A Rustecka, A Lipińska-Opałka, J Żuber, P Murawski, K Bilska and W Woźniak

Chapter 6

Infantile haemangiomas—IR thermography in assessment

Infrared thermography allows the assessment of the temperature of haemangiomas and their size in metric units (by using special software). Because of the diversity of haemangiomas in terms of their location, the age of the children and the progress of the healing process (atrophy of the haemangioma), it seems that the comparison of the average temperatures between an area registered within haemangioma and an area registered within a symmetrical body part is the most reliable method to describe treatment efficacy.

Thermographic images were taken in 42 children with different types of haemangiomas (14 boys, 28 girls). The children were participating in the propranolol therapy program. Based on the length of treatment with propranolol the patients were divided into two groups:

Group I—seven children who were examined using infrared imaging before starting propranolol treatment or during the first follow-up visit (after six weeks of treatment).

Group II—28 children who were examined using infrared imaging after several months of propranolol treatment, usually successful treatment with regression of clinical symptoms.

Outcome: The differences in average temperatures between an area measured with the haemangioma and an area measured within a symmetrical body part or an area adjacent to the haemangioma were: group I 1.29 °C and in group II 0.47 °C. See figures 6.1–6.7 for examples of individual cases.

doi:10.1088/978-0-7503-1143-4ch6

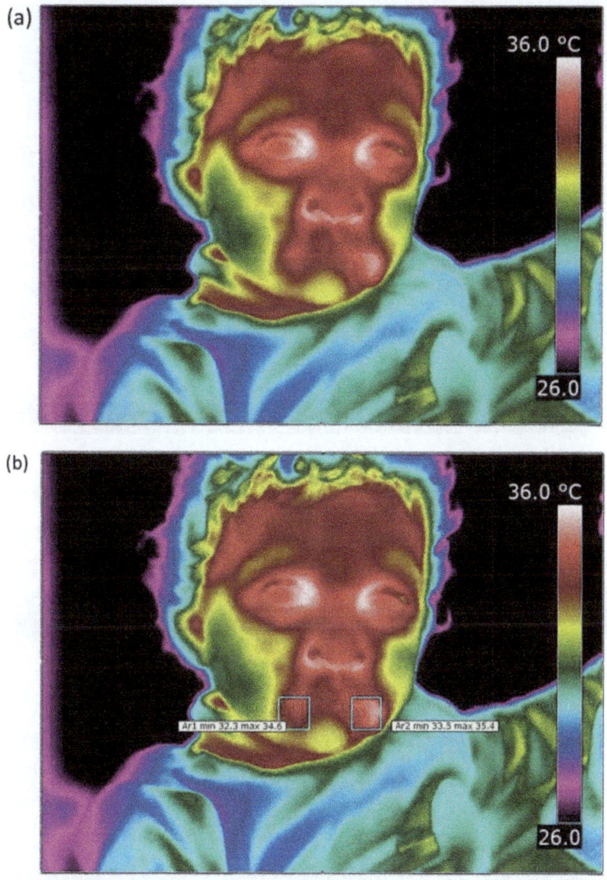

Figure 6.1. A 2.5-year-old girl with a haemangioma in the area of the left angle of the mouth. (*a*) Before treatment. (*b*) After 17 months of propranolol treatment. The difference in average temperatures in the area A2 within the haemangioma and the area A1 within a symmetric region is 1 °C.

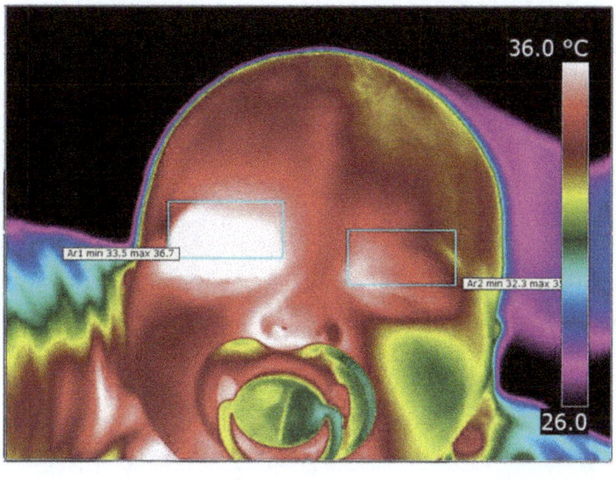

Figure 6.2. A two-month-old infant with a haemangioma of the right upper lid. The difference in average temperatures between symmetric areas was 1.5 °C.

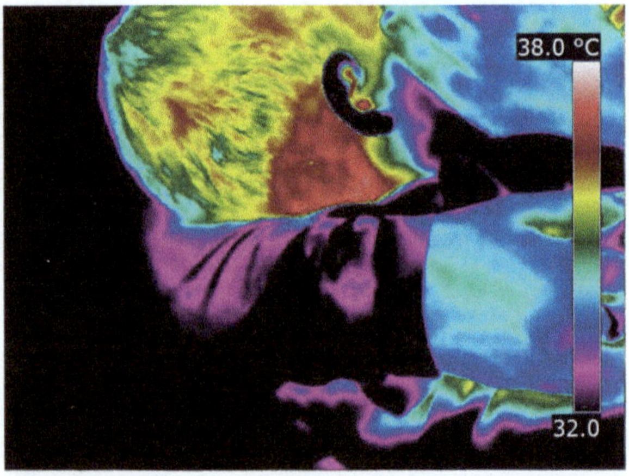

(a)

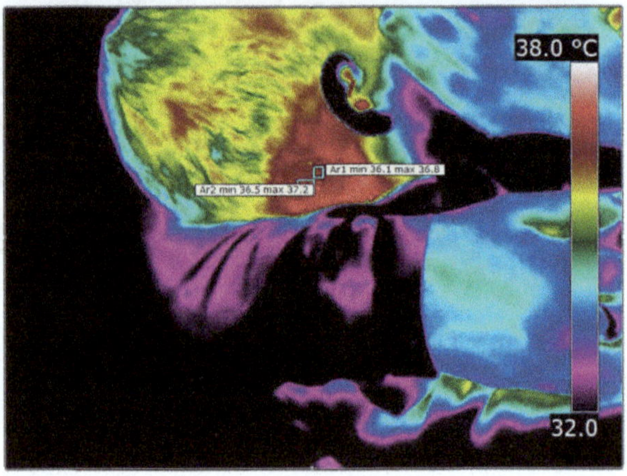

(b)

Figure 6.3. A nine-month-old infant with an infantile haemangioma of the skin in the area of the mastoid process. (*a*) Before treatment. (*b*) After four months of propranolol treatment. There are visible atrophic foci; the difference between average temperatures was 0.5 °C.

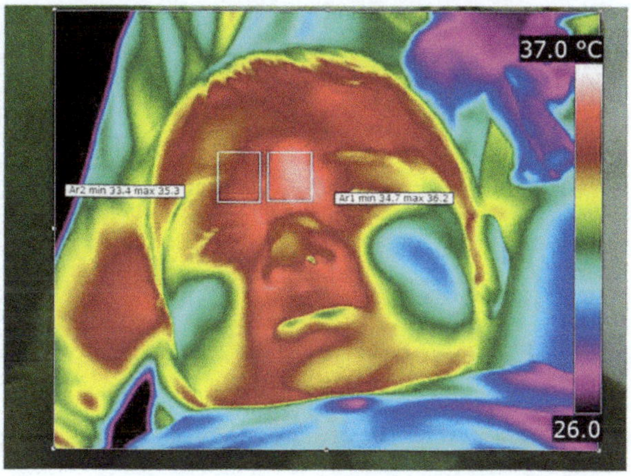

(a)

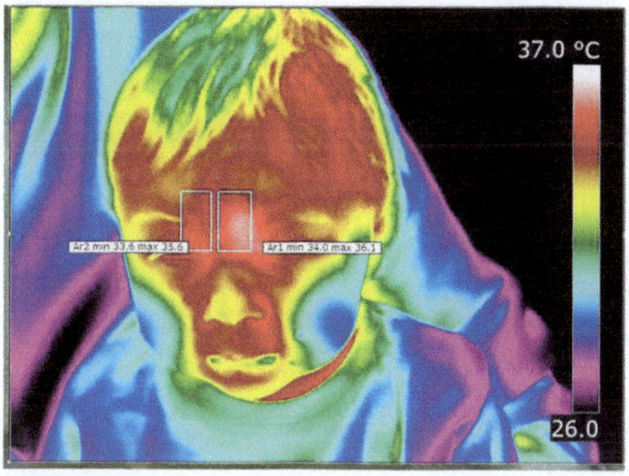

(b)

Figure 6.4. A 12-month-old boy with an infantile haemangioma of the skin in the area of the nasal bridge, on the left. (*a*) Before treatment—the difference between average temperatures was 1.3 °C. (*b*) After six weeks of propranolol treatment—the difference between average temperatures was 0.7 °C.

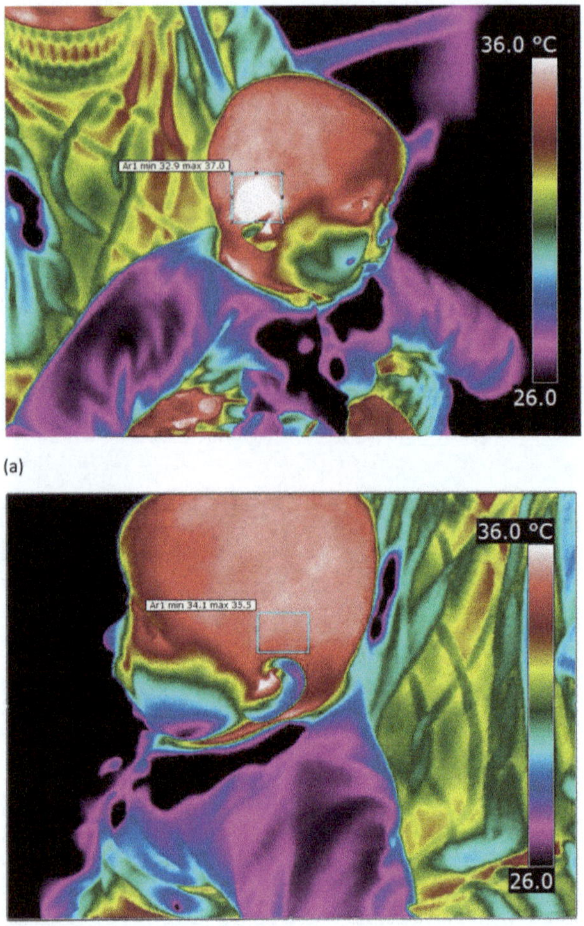

Figure 6.5. A three-month-old infant with an infantile haemangioma deforming the right auricle. The difference of average temperatures between an area within the haemangioma (*a*) and an area within a symmetric body part (*b*) was 1 °C.

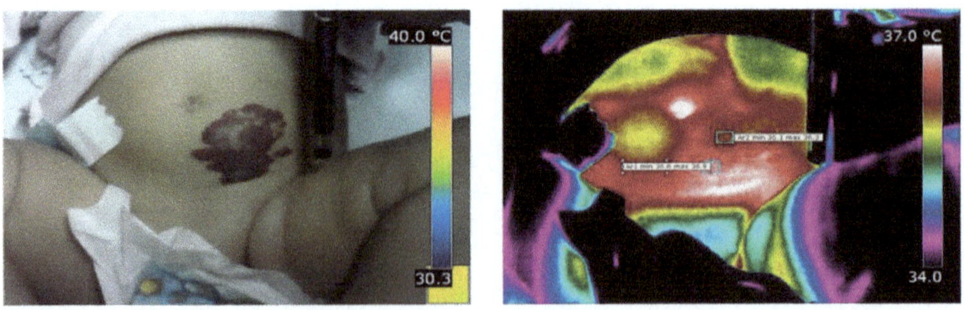

Figure 6.6. A 12-month-old girl with an infantile haemangioma. A1 is an area with high blood flow within the haemangioma determined by Doppler ultrasound, A2 is an area with marked atrophy of a highly vascularized region due to propranolol therapy. The average temperature in the area A1 = 36.8 °C, in the area A2 = 36.2 °C. The delta of the average temperatures was 0.6 °C.

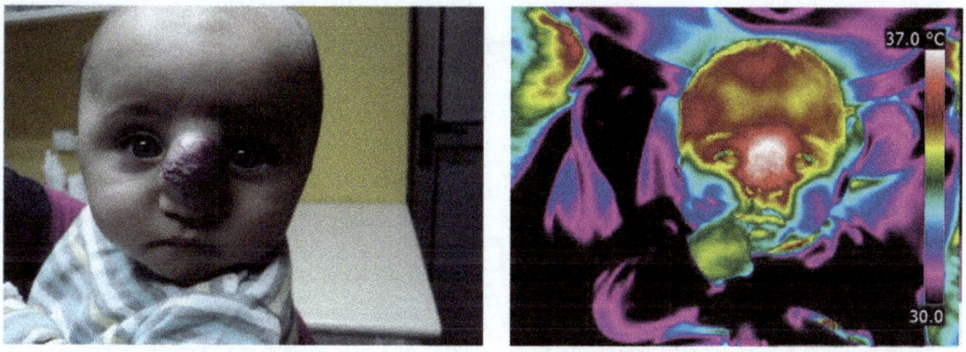

Figure 6.7. A seven-month-old boy with an inflamed and tender infantile haemangioma of the nose after four months of propranolol therapy. The tenderness of the haemangioma limited the use of Doppler ultrasound. Visual and thermographic evaluation allowed full control of the healing process.

IOP Publishing

Infrared Imaging
A casebook in clinical medicine
Costanzo Di Maria, Petros Perros, Jane Dickinson and John Allen

Chapter 7

Exploratory thermal and laser speckle contrast imaging measurements of eye inflammation in a case of thyroid eye disease

7.1 Description

TED is a thyroid-related condition that can affect the eyes of patients suffering from Graves' disease. Medical treatment of these patients is guided by identifying the disease phase, defined as *active* or *inactive*. Patients with active TED are given medical treatments. Medical treatment is ineffective in patients with inactive disease who may be best treated with surgery instead. At the same time, surgery is usually inappropriate during the active disease phase [1].

The current standard practice for determining disease phase in TED is by assessing the presence or absence of seven clinical signs of inflammation. One point is assigned for the presence of each sign and their sum forms the clinical activity score (CAS). A CAS value of at least 3 out of 7 is considered to indicate active disease. However, this method is subjective and can be misleading.

Microvascular imaging techniques such as TI [2] and LSCI [3] could have an important role in this clinical setting [4] by offering a more objective assessment tool.

7.2 Clinical presentation

A 38-year-old female patient attended our tertiary centre reporting symptoms of TED during the last 19 months. On clinical ophthalmological assessment she was found to have proptosis of 22 mm in the right eye and 20 mm in the left eye; the palpebral aperture was 9.5 mm on the right eye and 9.0 mm on the left eye; she had no diplopia or chemosis. Blood tests revealed increased level of free tri-iodothyronine (fT3) of 27.6 pmol L^{-1} (normal range 3.5–6.5 pmol L^{-1}); increased level of free thyroxine (fT4) of 58.8 pmol L^{-1} (normal range 9.5–21.5 pmol L^{-1}); and suppressed serum thyroid stimulating hormone of < 0.05 mU L^{-1} (normal range

0.3–4.7 mU L^{-1})—all consistent with hyperthyroidism. She scored a CAS value of 4 and was, therefore, diagnosed with active TED.

7.3 Investigations and procedures, diagnostic findings

Microvascular imaging was undertaken following our standard cool-room tissue inflammation study protocol and performed at our microvascular facility at Freeman Hospital. Subject preparation involved avoiding facial cosmetics, smoking and caffeine for at least 3 h before the test and resting for 30 min in the waiting area outside the measurement facility. The temperature of the measurement room was set to 18 °C. The patient acclimatized in the measurement room resting on the measurement couch for 10 min before performing imaging.

TI was performed using a FLIR SC300 thermal camera, which was powered up for at least 2 h prior to the measurement commencing. Skin emissivity was set to 0.98 [5]. LSCI was performed using a Moor Instruments FLPI2 scanner system. The exposure time was set to 20 ms and the time filter to 25 frames. Sample images are given in figure 7.1.

The thermal image was visualized and analysed using FLIR ThermaCAM Researcher Pro 2.8 software. Temperature was colour-coded with a 'rainbow' colour scale [5], across the range 32–36 °C. On TI, the region of interest comprising the hottest area of the eye and peri-orbital region had a mean temperature of 35.4 °C at

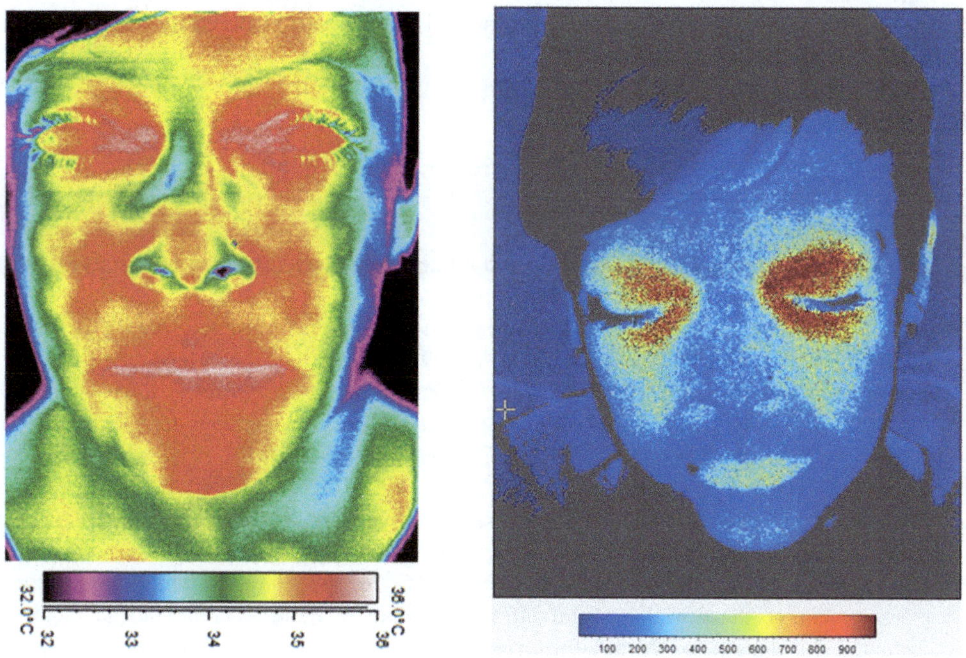

Figure 7.1. Sample thermal (left) and laser speckle contrast image (right) from a patient with active TED. The thermal image scale is given in degrees celsius. The laser speckle contrast image scale is given in AFU; the background level was set to 30 AFU. Laser speckle contrast image reproduced with permission from [4]. Copyright 2014 IOP Publishing.

both the right and left eye. This value was considerably higher than the reference mean temperature at the lateral orbit (34.0 °C at both the right and left lateral orbit).

The laser speckle contrast image was visualized and analysed using Moor Instruments FLPI Review V4.0 software. The flux was colour coded with a '256 colour palette 1' colour scale, across the range 0–1000 arbitrary flux units (AFU). On LSCI, the area comprising the upper and lower eyelid was found to have increased blood flux. The flux was 742 AFU at the right eye and 945 AFU at the left eye. This was about 3 and 4 times, respectively, the flux value at the forehead (246 AFU) taken as reference.

7.4 Brief discussion and conclusion

TI allows for rapid and non-invasive investigation of patients with TED. Specific temperature characteristics have been observed in this patient group, showing higher mean temperatures of the eye and peri-orbital region in comparison to healthy control subjects [6], reflecting the presence of inflammation. Simple mean temperature measurements have also been shown to decrease following methylprednisolone pulse therapy [7], which is consistent with the expected reduction of inflammation induced by the therapy. A more sophisticated, bespoke thermal image processing algorithm has also been proposed showing promising preliminary results in discriminating between patients with active and inactive disease [8].

This case study also shows the potential value of LSCI assessment of TED patients. The region of the eyes is characterized by high values of blood flux, which is indicative of tissue inflammation.

References

[1] Perros P, Neoh C and Dickinson 2009 Thyroid eye disease *Br. Med. J.* **338** b560

[2] Ring E F J and Ammer K 2012 Infrared thermal imaging in medicine *Physiol. Meas.* **33** R33–46

[3] Briers J D 2001 Laser Doppler, speckle and related techniques for blood perfusion mapping and imaging *Physiol. Meas.* **22** R35–66

[4] Allen J and Howell K 2014 Microvascular imaging: techniques and opportunities for clinical physiological measurements *Physiol. Meas.* **35** R91–141

[5] British Standards Institution 2010 *Medical Electrical Equipment. Particular Requirements for the Basic Safety and Essential Performance of Screening Thermographs for Human Febrile Temperature Screening* (London: BSI) BS EN 80601-part 2-59:2009

[6] Chang T C, Hsiao Y L and Liao S L 2008 Application of digital infrared thermal imaging in determining inflammatory state and follow-up effect of methylprednisolone pulse therapy in patients with Graves' ophthalmopat *Graefe's Arch. Clin. Exp. Ophthalmol.* **246** 45–9

[7] Shih S R, Li H Y, Hsiao Y L and Chang T C 2010 The application of temperature measurement of the eyes by digital infrared thermal imaging as a prognostic factor of methylprednisolone pulse therapy for Graves' ophthalmopathy *Acta Ophthalmol.* **88** e154–9

[8] Di Maria C, Allen J, Dickinson J, Neoh C and Perros P 2014 Novel thermal imaging analysis technique for detecting inflammation in thyroid eye disease *J. Clin. Endocrinol. Metabol.* **99** 4600–06

IOP Publishing

Infrared Imaging
A casebook in clinical medicine
B Kalicki, A Lipińska-Opałka and P Murawski

Chapter 8

Thermographic examination of a boy with an abscess near to the maxillary sinus

This chapter presents the possibility of a thermal imaging diagnosis of inflammatory conditions running within the sinuses.

The thermal imaging study was performed on a six-year-old boy admitted to the Department of Paediatrics, Nephrology and Allergy due to high fever and swelling of the right cheek and right lower eyelid. Physical examination showed the presence of an abscess around a molar tooth with purulent secretion. The thermal imaging study showed the temperature difference in symmetrical parts of the face—there was a hyperthermic area in the right maxillary sinus projection. After 3 d of antibiotic treatment, the oedema decreased substantially, which correlates well with the infrared image, figure 8.1.

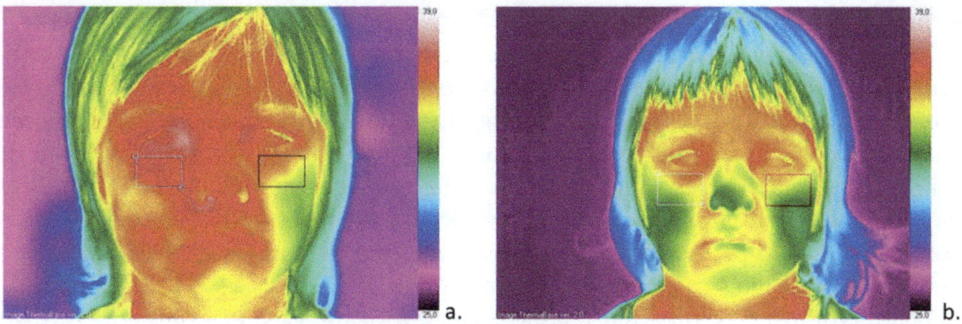

Figure 8.1. Thermography of patient's face. (*a*) Before treatment—the average temperature of the right cheek was 367 °C. (*b*) After 3 d of therapy—the average temperature of the right cheek was 34.3 °C. The temperature difference in the inflamed area before and after treatment was 2.4 °C.

doi:10.1088/978-0-7503-1143-4ch8

IOP Publishing

Infrared Imaging
A casebook in clinical medicine
Ricardo Vardasca, Liliana Esteves, Marco Rebelo and Joaquim Gabriel

Chapter 9

Malignant melanoma characterization with thermal and visual imaging

According to the World Health Organization, between 2 and 3 million non-melanoma skin cancers and 132 000 melanoma skin cancers occur globally each year. One in every three cancers diagnosed is a skin cancer. Thus, it is necessary to find new cost-effective tools that can contribute to early diagnosis or treatment assessment.

This medical imaging method was used for the physiological characterization of skin neoplasms in 58 patients. The images were recorded using a FLIR A325sc thermal camera (with a resolution of 320×240, a precision of 70 mK and an accuracy of ±2% of overall reading). The thermal images were recorded in an acclimatized room at 21 °C and a relative humidity of <50%, the subject was placed 80 cm away from the camera, which was mounted on a tripod (figure 9.1), and had acclimatized for 15 min before the recording.

Examples of visual and thermal images per type of skin neoplasm are given in figure 9.2, showing the benign lesions seborrheic keratosis, actinic keratosis and melanocytic nuvi, and the malignant lesions of basal cell carcinoma, squamous cell carcinoma and melanoma. Figure 9.3 shows the results of the quantitative analysis resulting from drawing two rectangular regions of interest over the neoplasm and calculating the thermal symmetry. It can be seen that from a diagnostic perspective the proposed method demonstrates the feasibility of identifying malignant cases (squamous cell carcinoma and basal cell carcinoma).

The relationship of different characteristics with the type of skin neoplasm was assessed and it was found that age, gender, body mass index and skin Sun sensitivity

doi:10.1088/978-0-7503-1143-4ch9

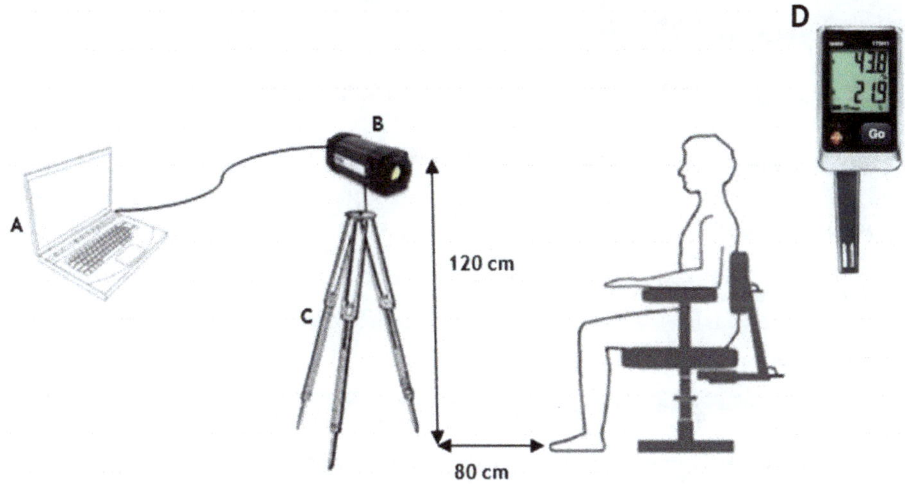

Figure 9.1. The capture set up for skin neoplasm thermal recording (*A*: laptop; *B*: thermal camera; *C*: tripod; and *D*: environmental variables meter).

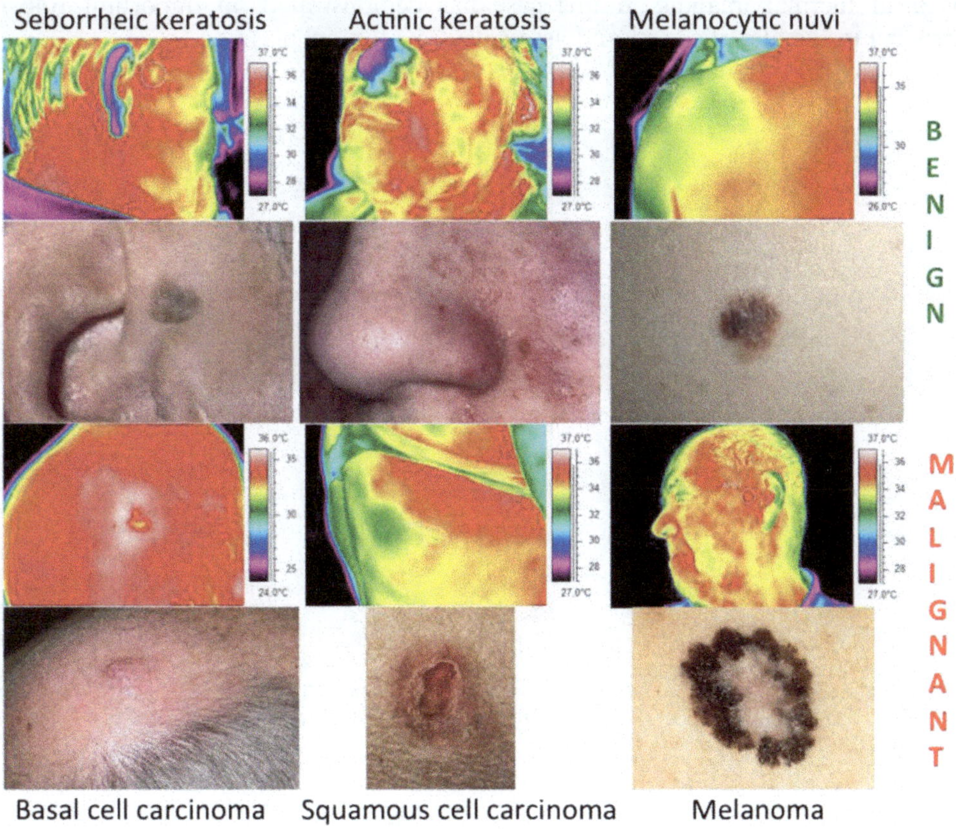

Figure 9.2. Examples of visual and thermal images of the different types of benign and malignant skin neoplasms.

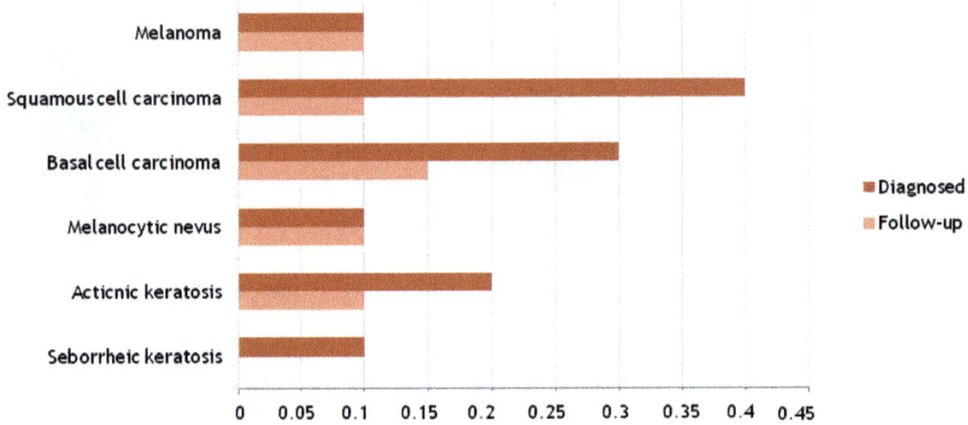

Figure 9.3. Thermal symmetry values obtained for the different skin neoplasms.

are related to skin temperature ($p < 0.05$). It was therefore possible, through a measure of thermal symmetry, to distinguish benign from malignant skin cancers. Medical thermal imaging in this case has demonstrated an important role in assisting in the identification and assessment of skin neoplasms.

IOP Publishing

Infrared Imaging
A casebook in clinical medicine

Anna Jung, Bolesław Kalicki, Janusz Żuber, Lech Gawron, Radosław Różycki, Andrzej Stankiewicz and Piotr Murawski

Chapter 10

Thermographic monitoring of ophthalmic surgery—extraction of a cataract

Cataract surgery was performed using phaco-emulsification and was divided into several stages: local anaesthesia, pulsed emulsification of the nucleus lens and implantation of a post-camera intra-ocular lens. Thermograms were recorded before and during surgery and 15, 30 and 60 min after (see figures 10.1–10.14).

Research thermography was performed with the infrared camera ThermaCAM SC1000. The requirements and conditions for clinical thermography were established.

The images were analysed using the specialized software 'Image ThermaBase'.

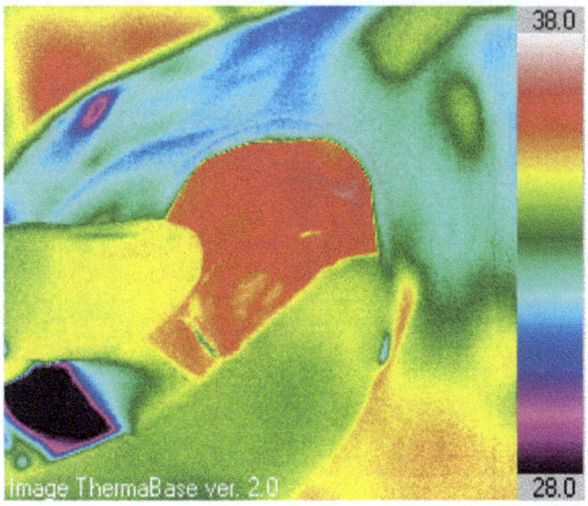

Figure 10.1. Thermogram of the right eye before surgery.

doi:10.1088/978-0-7503-1143-4ch10

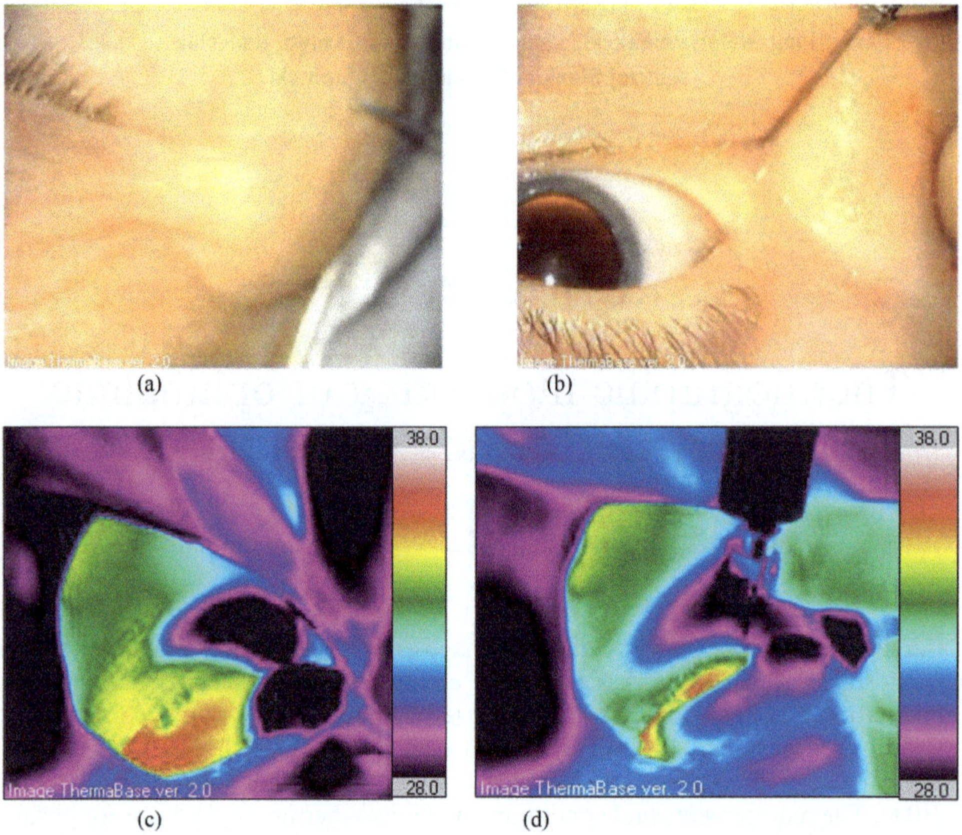

Figure 10.2. Visual images and thermograms of the right eye. (*a*), (*b*) Visual images corresponding to (*c*) and (*d*). (*c*) After anaesthesia of the eyelid: T_{min} = 25.1 °C, T_{max} = 36.3 °C. (*d*) During retrobulbar anaesthesia: T_{min} = 26.6 °C, T_{max} = 36.1 °C.

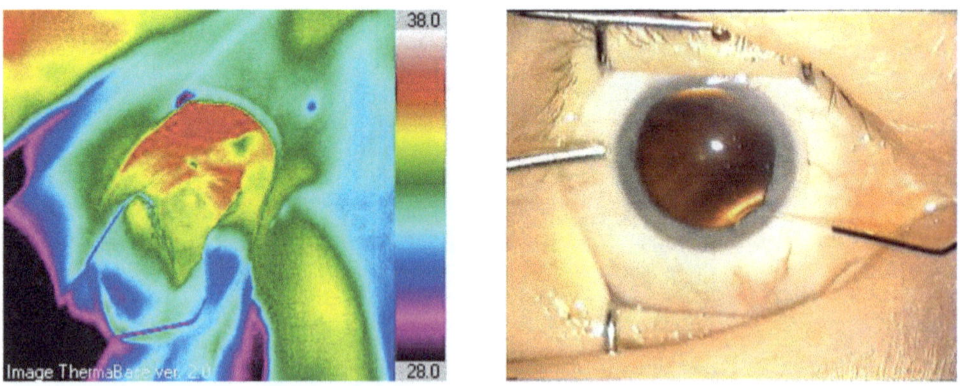

Figure 10.3. Thermal image of the right eye after local and retro-ocular anaesthesia. A decrease of the value of the temperature on the eye's surface of 4.2 °C was observed.

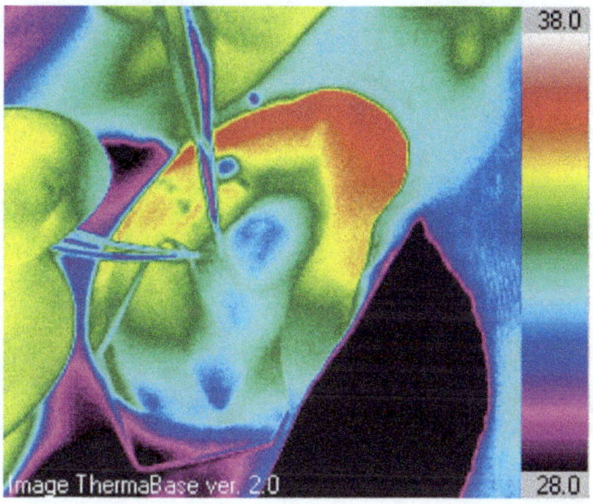

Figure 10.4. Thermal image of the right eye after moistening the eye surface (0.9% NaCl) at the beginning of the surgery.

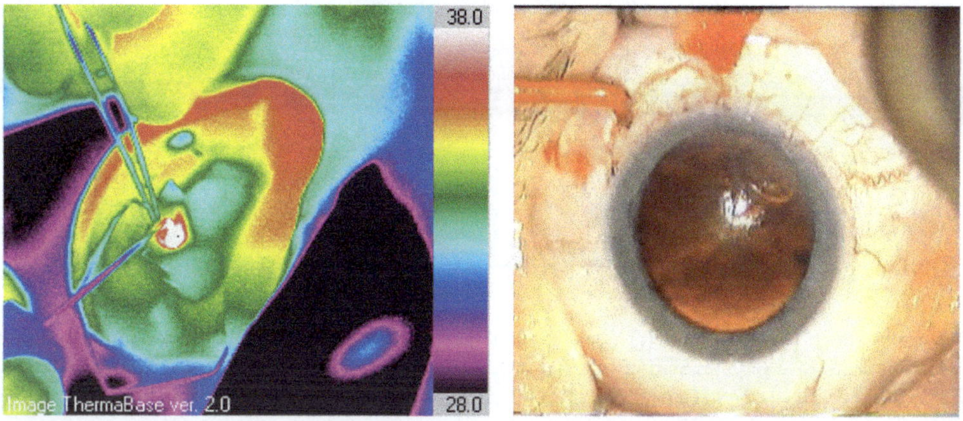

Figure 10.5. Thermal image of the right eye during diathermal coagulation. A local increase of temperature to 64 °C for a few seconds was observed.

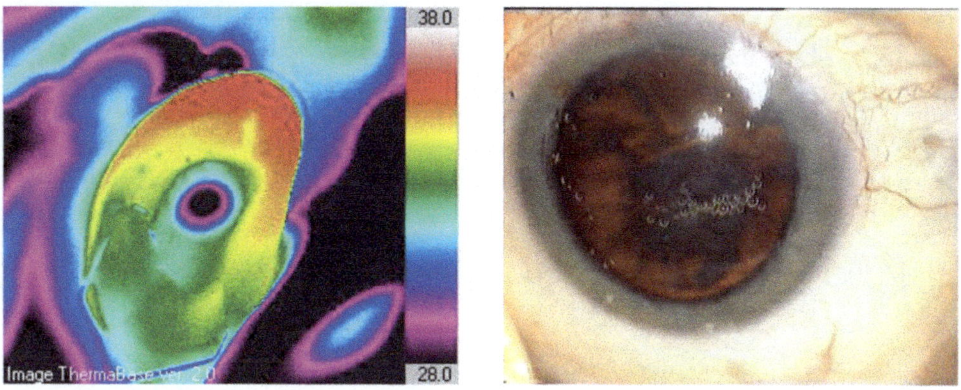

Figure 10.6. Thermal end visual image of the right eye in the next stage of surgery. The view after opening an anterior chamber and using a visco-elastic substance.

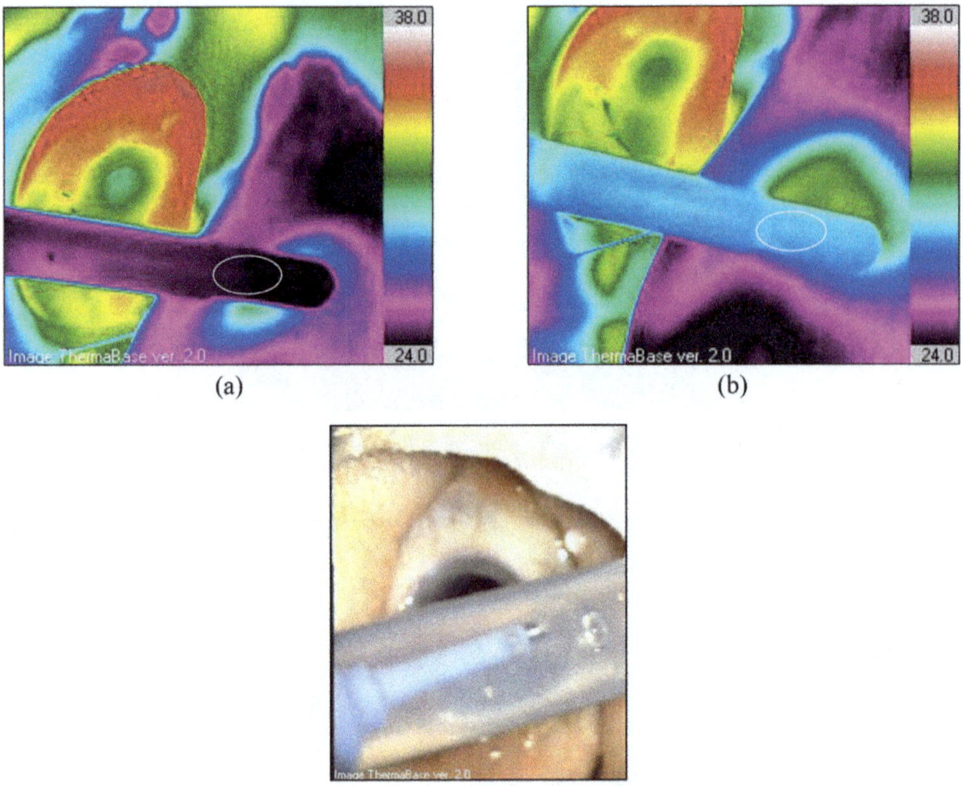

Figure 10.7. (*a*), (*b*) Thermograms. (*c*) Visual image of the ultrasonic probe for phaco-emulsification during the test before cataract surgery. (*a*) Start of test: $T_{min} = 23.6$ °C, $T_{max} = 24.6$ °C, median = 24.1 °C. (*b*) End of test: $T_{min} = 27.0$ °C, $T_{max} = 27.9$ °C, median = 27.5 °C. $\Delta T_{max} = 3.3$ °C.

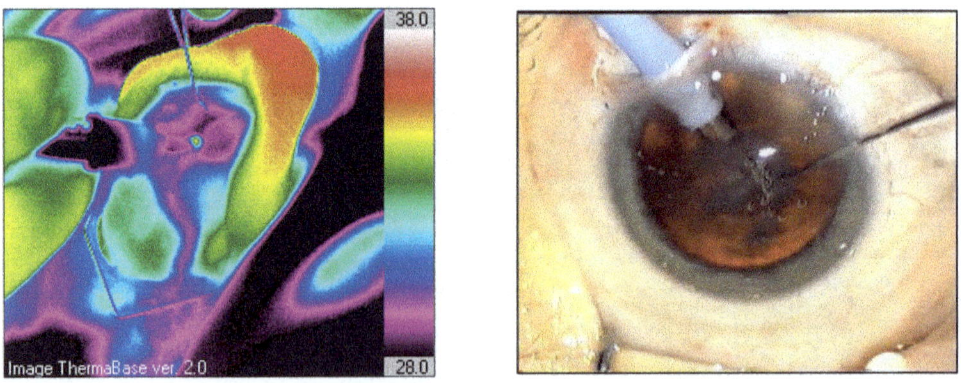

Figure 10.8. Thermogram and visual image during phaco-emulsification. The local increase in temperature was only 0.6 °C.

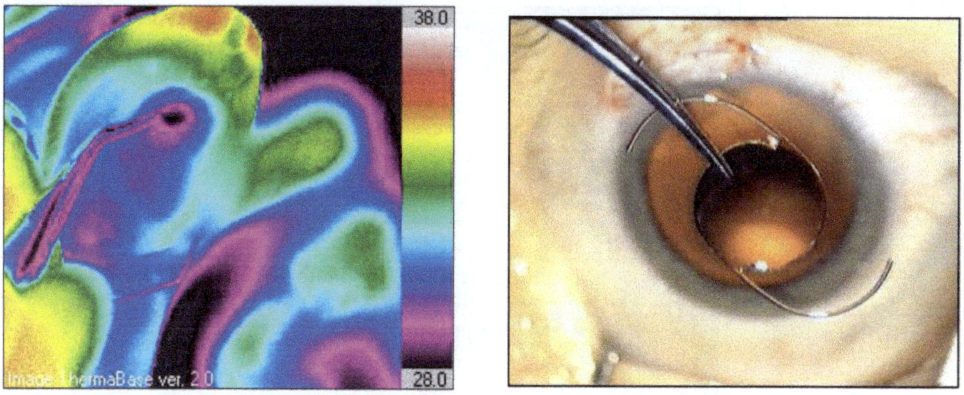

Figure 10.9. Thermogram and visual image of the artificial lens before implantation. $T_{avg} = 28.3$ °C, SD = 0.3.

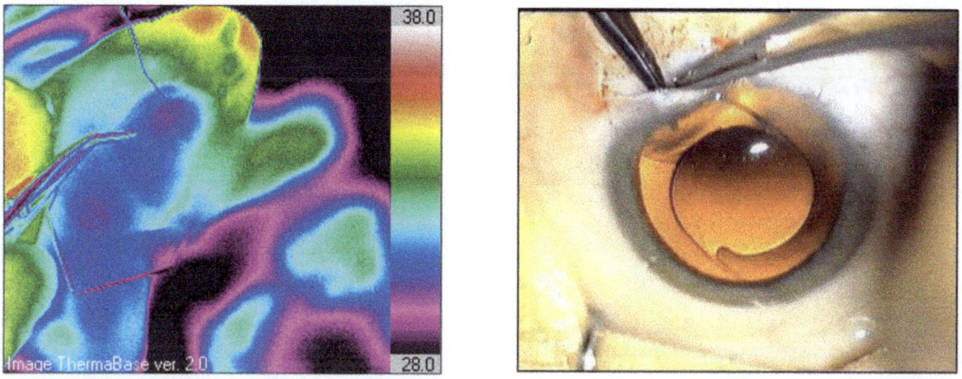

Figure 10.10. Thermogram and visual image after implantation the lens of the post-camera.

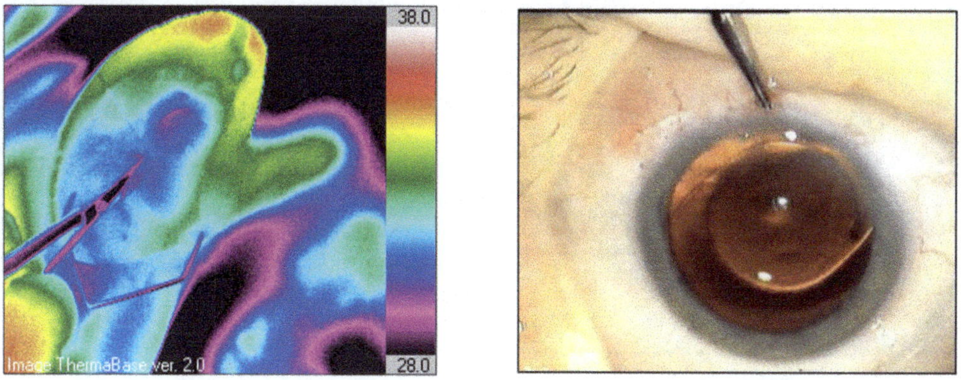

Figure 10.11. Thermogram and visual image during the last stage of surgery.

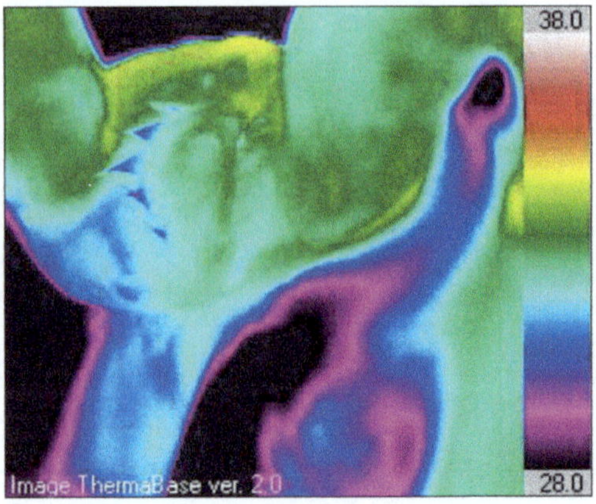

Figure 10.12. Thermogram 15 min after surgery. An increase in temperature of 1.2 °C on the eye's surface was observed.

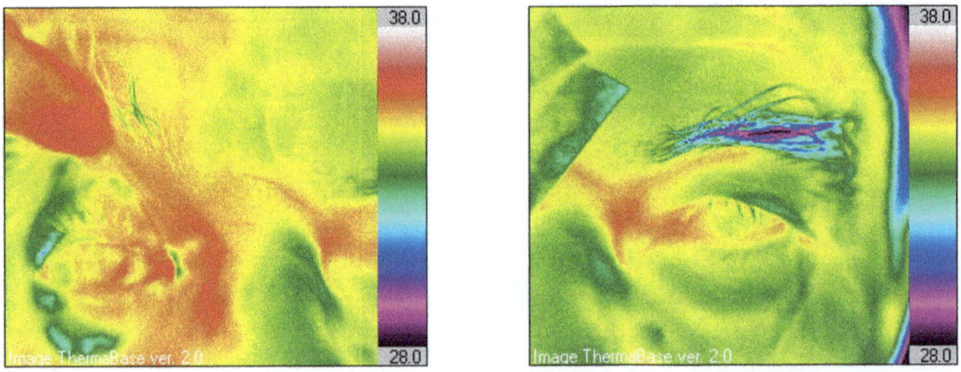

(a) (b)

Figure 10.13. Thermograms 30 min after surgery and 60 min after anaesthesia. Changes in the temperature in the area of local eyelid anaesthesia were observed. (*a*) Right eye after surgery. (*b*) Left eye (for comparison).

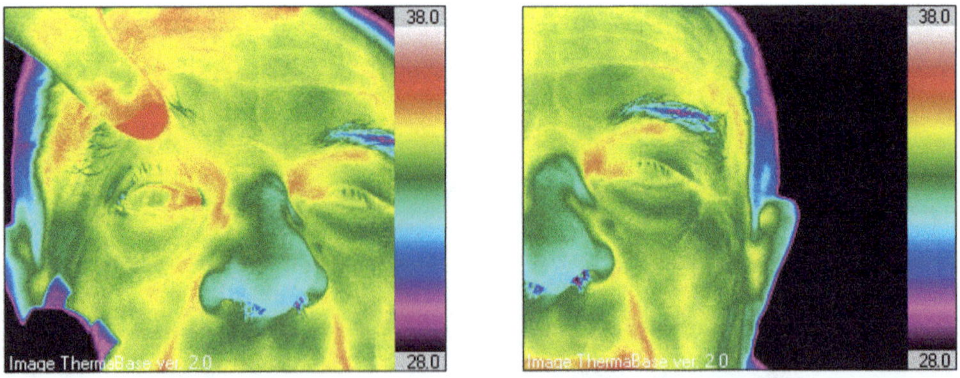

(a) (b)

Figure 10.14. Thermograms 60 min after surgery and 90 min after anaesthesia. (*a*) Right eye after surgery. (*b*) Left eye (for comparison).

10.1 Conclusions

During cataract surgery an increase of the temperature was observed only during surgical diathermy. The increase was local and of a few seconds' duration.

During the phaco-emulsification the temperature of the probe increased by 0.6 °C and achieved the temperature of the surrounding tissues. This procedure was therefore shown not to damage the tissues.

Chapter 11

Application of thermal imaging in the diagnosis of inflammatory changes of nasal sinusitis

The nasal cavity, along with the nasal sinuses, is a space in which it is important to keep a constant temperature. The physiological activities of the nose are closely connected to the air flow through the nose, creating the only physiological respiratory tract [1]. In the case of high temperature of the surrounding air, the breathing path through the mouth is used. The same also occurs in cases of anatomical abnormality of the upper respiratory tract and lungs, circulatory system diseases and during exercise. But it should be emphasized that only breathing through the nose ensures the proper thermal cycling of the air inspired from the environment. Warming of the inspired air occurs due to heat transfer from the blood circulating in the vessels of subcutaneous tissues, mostly in the cavernous plexuses in the posterior nares. The warmed air reaches a temperature of 32 °C–34 °C independent of the temperature of the breathed air [1]. The process of warming the inspired air can be investigated in the study of the heat emission registered by a thermal imaging camera [1]. Under physiological conditions it assumes a symmetrical picture in both nostrils with regularly rising temperature from the anterior to posterior nares. There are also two other factors which determine the proper physiological activities of the nasal sinuses, namely ventilation and permeability. Ventilation depends on maintaining the proper width and permeability of the fissures connecting the sinuses with the nasal cavities. Permeability is affected by the secretion of mucus and its transport outside the sinuses. The whole process can be demonstrated by thermographic examination. Under inappropriate conditions the symmetry of the thermographic picture can be disturbed. The standardization and objective measurement of thermal changes has paved the way for the use of large scale thermal imaging in the diagnosis of inflammatory focus [2]. The possibility of differentiating the aetiology of the mucous membrane changes of allergic or inflammatory origin are of particular interest and value in clinical practice.

doi:10.1088/978-0-7503-1143-4ch11

The thermographic evaluation of cases with a range of inflammatory changes in the area of the paranasal sinuses was compared with radiological images (see figures 11.1–11.4). Thermographic evaluation also provided non-invasive monitoring of the pathological process, eliminating the need for computed tomography.

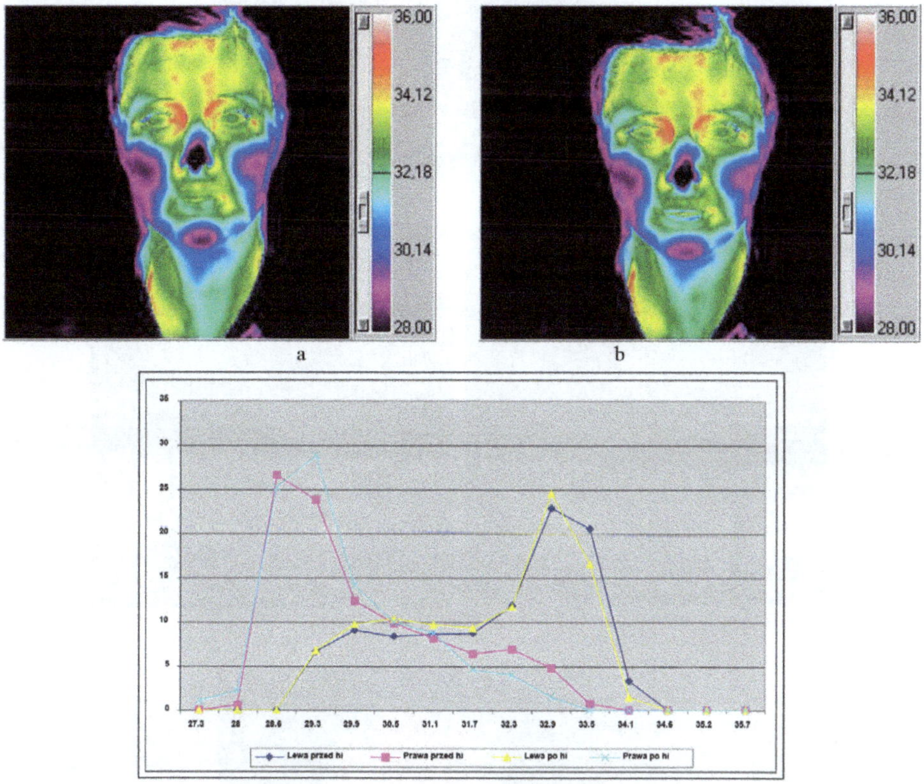

Figure 11.1. Thermograms and a histogram of a patient (KI) with left maxillary sinusitis: (*a*) before hyperventilation; (*b*) after hyperventilation; and (*c*) the histogram.

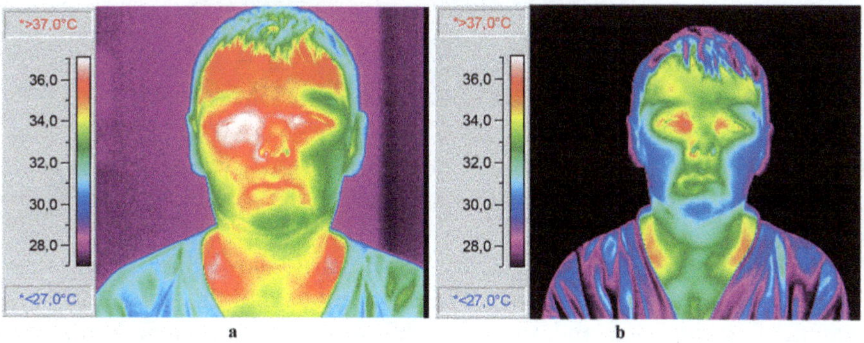

Figure 11.2. Thermograms of a patient (RM) with right ethmoiditis and bilateral sinusitis (*a*) before treatment and (*b*) after treatment.

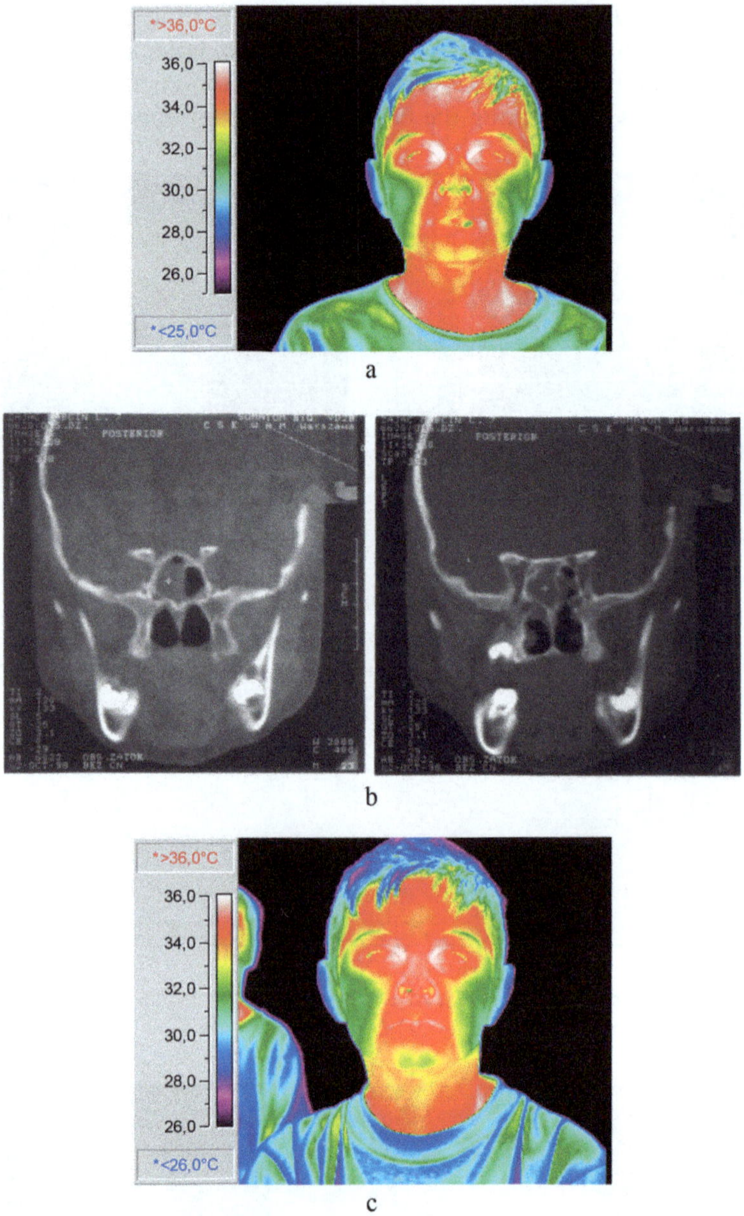

Figure 11.3. Thermograms and computed tomography images of a patient (ZM) with ethmoiditis and right maxillary sinusitis: (*a*), (*b*) before treatment and (*c*) after treatment.

The hyperventilation test proved to be of particular value. When there was increased air flow through the nasal cavities, an increase in the temperature gradient between the healthy area and the inflamed area was observed. Similarly, more information was obtained from a dynamic examination using the hyperventilation test, used in out-patient follow-ups. Temperature differences were observed between

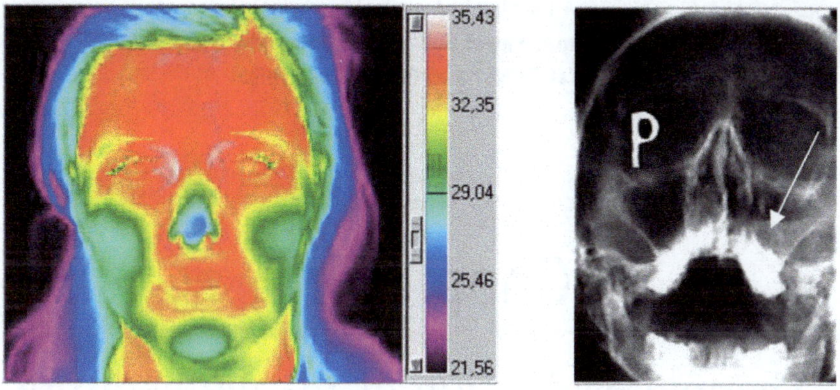

Figure 11.4. Thermogram and radiogram of a patient (KI) with left-sided maxillary sinusitis.

the healthy area and the area after inflammation, which were not registered by the statistical investigation.

There have been a few papers on the thermographic evaluation of the inflammatory changes in nasal sinuses. For example, the authors of [3] emphasize the asymmetry of the thermovisual image in the case of unilateral inflammatory changes. Accordingly to Wojaczyńska-Stanek [4] the sensitivity of detection of inflammatory changes using this method is about 80%.

During the examination of the patient KI (figure 11.1) a hyperthermal image in the area of the orbit and the maxillary sinus on the left side was recorded. A smaller hyperthermal focus was also observed in the area of the left maxillary sinus. The temperature gradient observed between the hyperthermal area and the surrounding tissues reached 3 °C.

Slightly lower temperature gradients have been registered in the mucosa of the collateral cavities in oedema which have an allergic basis. The hyperthermal areas are sometimes slightly smaller and more lateral [1]. The thermographic images presented are not sharp but show poorly defined borders of the hypo- and hyperthermal areas. Nevertheless, they shows the clinical value of thermographic investigation in differentiating an inflammatory state of the nasal cavities from mucosal oedema in cavities of an allergic origin.

References

[1] Seppey M, Hessler C, Brucker M, Savary M and Pecoud A 1993 Facial thermography during nasal provocation test with histamine and alergen *Allergy* **48** 314

[2] Fujimasa I 1995 Standardisation of techniques for thermal image testing: the current situation *Biomed. Theromol.* **15** 63–8

[3] Melnitzky P, Schaltemuller T and Ammer K 1997 Thermography in sinusitus patients *Eur. J. Thermol.* **7** 67

[4] Wojaczynska-Stanek K, Marszat E, Emich-Widera E and Dermolińska B 1997 Thermographic images of faces of children with allergies *Eur. J. Thermol.* **7** 67

IOP Publishing

Infrared Imaging

A casebook in clinical medicine

Stanisław Żmuda, Paweł Zaborowski, Mirosław Dąbrowski, Rafał Dulski and Cezary Pogorzelski

Chapter 12

Thermal evaluation of the temperature distribution in the oral cavity during dental operations

Caries is the most frequent disease of the mouth. Treatment uses mechanical tools or lasers to remove the surface of the damaged hard tissues. The re-forming of tissues which have been removed is performed using a base material and a filler. Most current stomatological materials are light hardened. For polymerization of these materials halogen lamps are commonly used. Investigations have shown a significant temperature increase during polymerization which may have a destructive influence on the dental pulp. Since thermal imaging only shows the superficial temperature disposition, comparative spot temperature measurements using thermoelements were used to evaluate temperatures within the filling material (see figures 12.1–12.4).

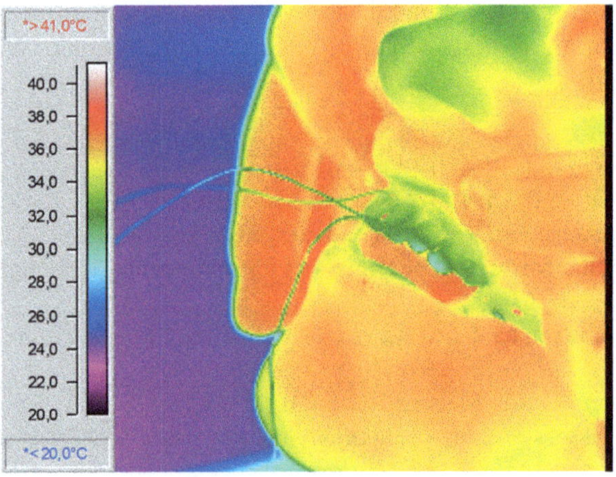

Figure 12.1. The conditions before caries healing (with a thermocouple installed). A thermal image of teeth 11 and 21.

doi:10.1088/978-0-7503-1143-4ch12

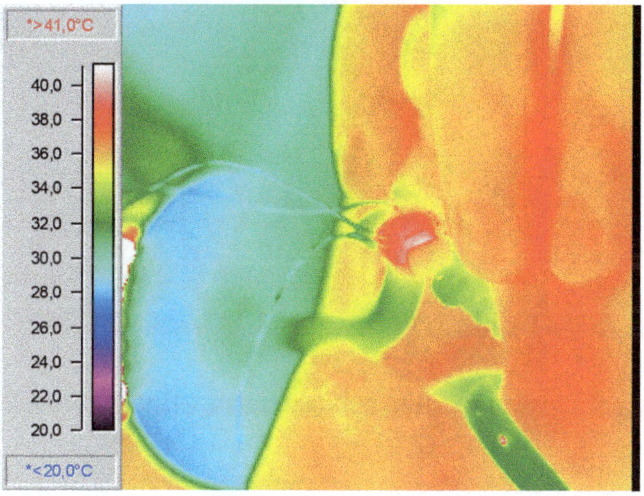

Figure 12.2. Polymerization process of a base material layer after caries preparation. The temperature distribution on the surface of tooth 21 allows the evaluation of the level of temperature increase. The tissues of the neighbouring teeth have a physiological temperature.

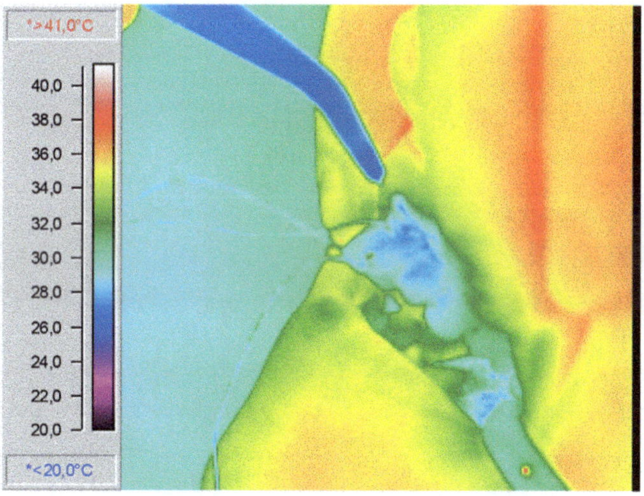

Figure 12.3. Drying process after the etching and rinsing phases. The temperature decrease of the teeth can be seen.

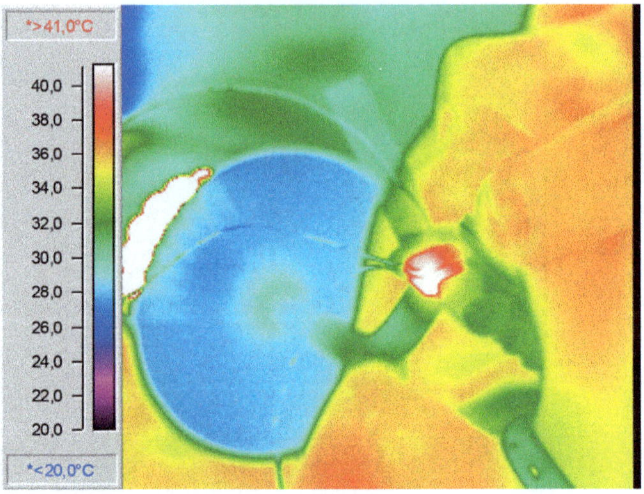

Figure 12.4. Filling material polymerization phase. The temperature increase of tooth 21 is higher compared to the curing phase of the base material.

IOP Publishing

Infrared Imaging
A casebook in clinical medicine
John Allen and Grainne Gorman

Chapter 13

Thermographic assessment of the presence of fatty tumours in myoclonic epilepsy with ragged red fibres

13.1 Description

MERRF is a rare maternally inherited multisystem disorder presenting most commonly with myopathy, cardiomyopathy, progressive myoclonic seizures, ataxia and hearing loss. Up to 80% of MERRF cases are due to the m.8344A>G in the *MT-TK* gene encoding tRNALys. Lipomatous MERRF is a relatively recently described sub-phenotype of this rare mitochondrial disease. The precise cellular mechanisms underpinning lipoma formation are unknown [1].

This case study sought to characterize the thermal and metabolic profiles of these benign adipose tumours in a patient with multiple lipoma secondary to MERRF.

13.2 Clinical presentation

We investigated a woman with multiple symmetrical lipomas in the neck due to the m.8344A>G MERRF mutation.

13.3 Investigations and procedures, diagnostic findings

The imaging included standard microvascular imaging by the author JA at the Microvascular Diagnostics measurement facility at Freeman Hospital with thermal imaging of the upper torso with anterior and posterior views using a thermal imaging camera (FLIR Systems SC300) [2].

For the thermal imaging the patient followed the pre-imaging protocol instructions which included avoiding any smoking, caffeinated substances and talc/creams on the skin on the day of their test. They arrived at the hospital and were acclimatized for 20 min in the temperature controlled room for the imaging (at 23 °C) [3].

doi:10.1088/978-0-7503-1143-4ch13

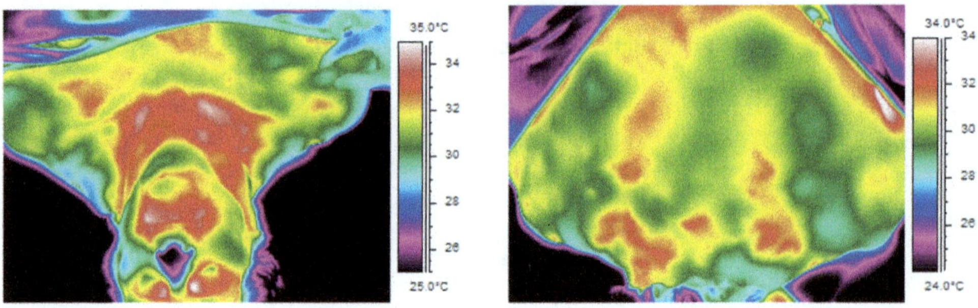

(a) (b)

Figure 13.1. Anterior and posterior views of the patient with MERRF. In (*a*) a cool area at the site of a palpable lipoma as located between the fingers of the clinician. In contrast, image (*b*) shows striking regions of local heat compared to surrounding tissue and associated with active lipoma tissue.

Images were then displayed using a 'rainbow scale' over a 10° C range with dedicated image processing software (FLIR ThermaCam Researcher, skin emissivity = 0.97). In figure 13.1 two distinct features can be seen at visible palpable lipoma tissue margins when compared to surrounding tissue: local hot areas of tissue typically elevated by 1–2 °C and also marginally cooler areas.

13.4 Brief discussion and conclusion

Thermal imaging has the potential to quickly and non-invasively study lipoma tissue in patients with MERRF. Further research is needed to assess a range of patients with MERRF and compare the local hot and cold spots with clinical and histological findings. Such further research could help us to understand the significance of the increased heat production that can be observed in this patient group.

References

[1] Cohen B H 2013 Neuromuscular and systemic presentations in adults: diagnoses beyond MERRF and MELAS *Neurotherapeutics* **10** 227–42

[2] Ring E F J and Ammer K 2012 Infrared thermal imaging in medicine *Physiol. Meas.* **33** R33–46

[3] Allen J and Howell K J 2014 Clinical microvascular imaging: techniques and opportunities for clinical physiological measurements *Physiol. Meas.* **35** R91–141

IOP Publishing

Infrared Imaging
A casebook in clinical medicine
B Kalicki, A Jung, A Rustecka, A Lipińska-Opałka, A Koszycka and W Stankiewicz

Chapter 14

Tietze's syndrome and the role of infrared imaging in the differential diagnosis of acute chest pain in adolescents

Tietze's syndrome is an inflammatory process affecting one or more chondrosternal joints of the anterior chest. It is characterized by painful and tender swelling, with a predilection to the upper ribs (figure 14.1). The diagnosis is made on clinical grounds after exclusion of other conditions presenting with acute chest pain. Physicians are still looking for simple, safe and non-invasive diagnostic methods to support the diagnosis of Tietze's syndrome. Infrared thermography, an innovative diagnostic method, can be used to diagnose Tietze's costochondritis. Thermography allows one to see variations in temperature of the skin and organs caused by an ongoing inflammatory process (figure 14.2).

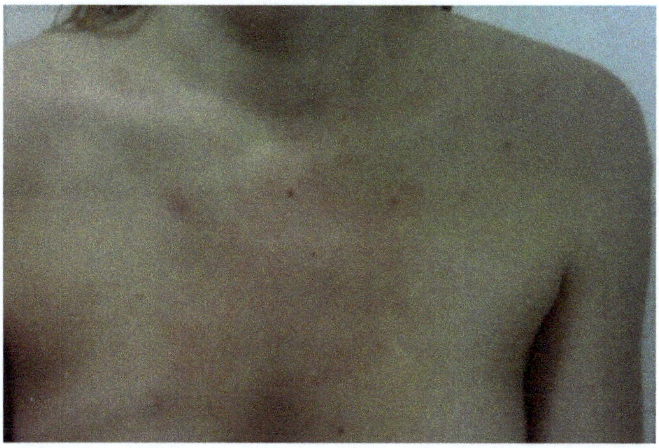

Figure 14.1. A visual image of changes observed during the physical examination of the patient.

doi:10.1088/978-0-7503-1143-4ch14

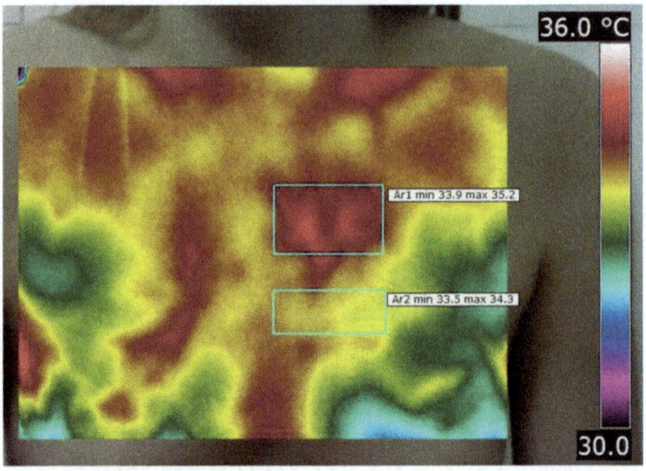

Figure 14.2. Thermographic image of the same area presented above. Because of the possibility of increased participation of infrared radiation in the region of the vascular trunk, area A1 was compared to area A2, located below the swelling of the chest wall. The difference between A1 and A2 was 1.4 °C for minimal temperatures and 0.9 °C for maximal temperatures.

IOP Publishing

Infrared Imaging
A casebook in clinical medicine
Bartosz Rustecki, Marcin Możański, Weronika Machura, Jakub Klimkiewicz, Anna Jung and Bolesław Kalicki

Chapter 15

Thoracic vertebral block—the technique of injecting local anaesthetic

Thoracic paravertebral block (TPVB) is a technique of injecting local anaesthetic in the paravertebral space where spinal nerves emerge from intervertebral foramina. It is effective in treating acute and chronic pain of unilateral origin from the chest and abdomen including post-operative pain [1–5]. When used peri-operatively TPVB provides excellent pain relief with pulmonary function preservation and great hemodynamic stability [6–8].

When properly injected local anaesthetic blocks pain stimuli as well as creating a sympathetic block with skin vessel diastole. This increases skin blood flow and makes the blocked region warmer. The first attempt to use infrared imaging to evaluate the efficacy of paravertebral block for breast surgery was performed by our research team in 2014.

A 66-year-old woman (156 cm, 80 kg, BMI 32) with chronic obstructive pulmonary disease, chronic right heart failure, hypertension and obesity, on long term oxygen therapy was presented for elective mastectomy due to cancer. The severe comorbidities raised concerns about post-operative pain control using opioid analgesics. The TPVB was chosen as part of a multimodal anaesthetic management.

The TPVB was performed using the multi-shot percutaneous technique. An FLIR i7 infrared camera was used to measure skin temperature changes 20 and 30 min after the TPVB to confirm adequate anaesthesia and the anaesthesia range (figures 15.1 and 15.2). The infrared photo showed an increase of the temperature readings in every marked region, as seen in figure 15.3. Light general anaesthesia was also used. There were no hemodynamic or pulmonary complications post-operatively. There was no need for rescue treatment with opioids. The TPVB in combination with light general anaesthesia created excellent conditions for the breast surgery procedure [7].

doi:10.1088/978-0-7503-1143-4ch15

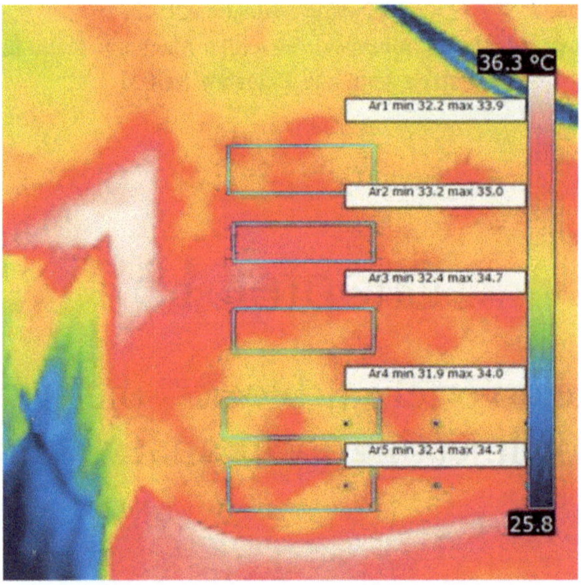

Figure 15.1. Photo taken before TPVB [7].

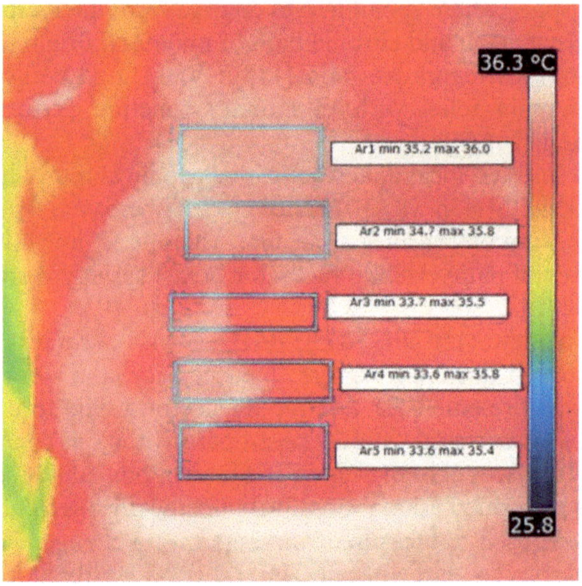

Figure 15.2. Photo taken 30 min after TPVB [7].

The promising results of using infrared scanning in this case lead us to use infrared technology in experimental research in an attempt to evaluate two techniques of TPVB: the one-shot technique and the multi-shot technique. The multi-shot technique, in theory, provides more complete anaesthesia, but takes longer to carry out and creates a higher risk of complications as two or three separate injections are performed.

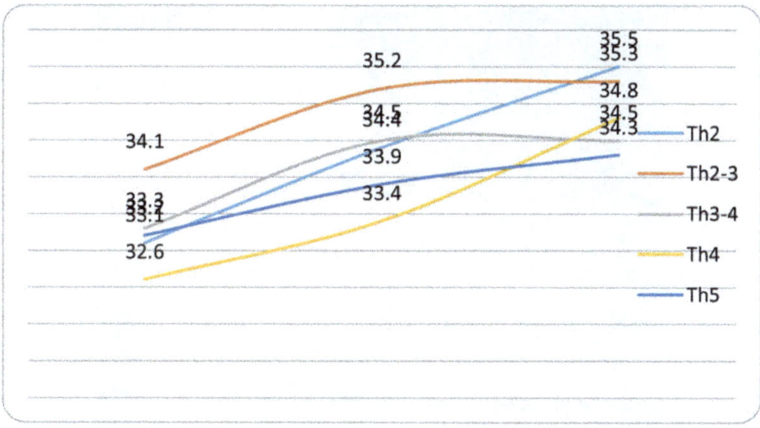

Figure 15.3. Temperature changes in Celsius count (x) at check points: 1—before TPVB; 2—20 min after TPVB; 3—30 min after TPVB [7].

Patients presented for elective mastectomy were enrolled and randomized into two groups: the first group (O) ($n = 17$) who received one-shot of TPVB at Th3 level and the second group (M) ($n = 13$) who received a multi-shot TPVB at the Th2, Th4 and Th6 levels. We used 0.5% *ropivacaine* with 0.1 mg of *fentanyl* in the total volume of $0.3\,\text{ml kg}^{-1}$ IBW (ideal body weight). IBW was calculated using the formula: height (cm) – 105. In the M group the total volume of local anaesthetic was divided into three equal parts [8].

Before and 20 min after the TPVB we took infrared photos of the breast region with an FLIR i7 camera for temperature change detection in order to capture the effects of the sympathetic blockade. The marked region was divided into three parts—the upper, middle and lower part of the breast—to evaluate the changes of temperature in the corresponding dermatomes. We also attempted to check changes in armpit temperature, but that failed due to poor visualization of the armpit in the photos taken. When the photos had been taken general anaesthesia was administered using the standardized protocol. Blind investigators studied the pain scores post-operatively and the need for rescue analgesic during and peri-operatively [8].

In group M ($n = 13$) in the upper part of the marked region the temperature increased in six patients, while in both the middle and lowest parts it increased in nine patients. There was no temperature increase in three patients. Twice we observed the increase of the temperature in one marked region (once in the middle and once the in lower part). Another two patients had a temperature increase in two regions, the middle and the lower parts. In six patients we observed an increase of temperature in all checked regions of the breast. See figures 15.4 and 15.5 for examples [8].

In group O ($n = 17$) in the upper, lower and middle marking points the temperature increased in eight patients out of 17, respectively. There was no temperature elevation in seven patients. In eight patients we observed increases of temperature in at least two marked regions, including six patients for whom the temperature increased in all marked regions. In two patients the temperature only increased in one region, once in the upper and once in the lower part. See figures 15.6 and 15.7 for examples [8].

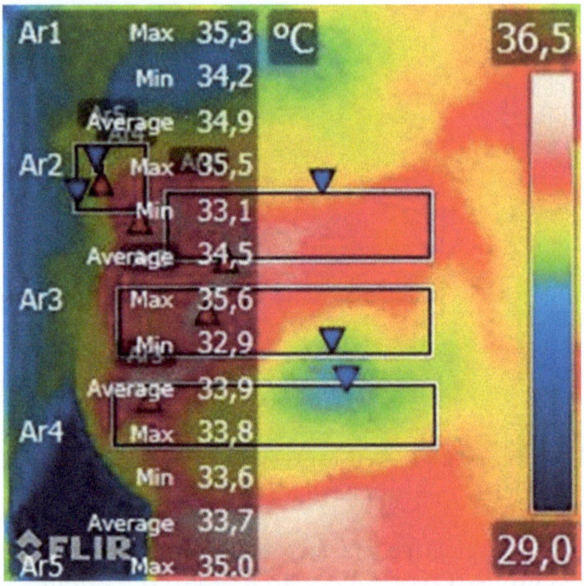

Figure 15.4. Infrared photo after analysis taken before analgesia, in the multi-shot group.

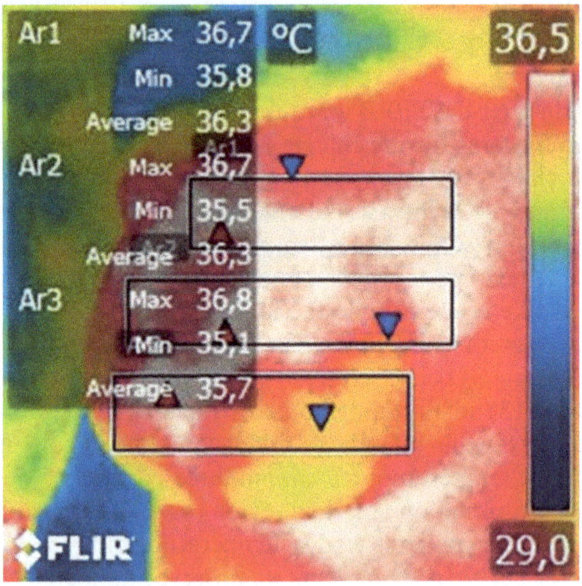

Figure 15.5. Infrared photo taken 20 min after TPVB in the multi-shot group.

We observed a lack of differences in drug usage during general anaesthesia and similar low pain levels after anaesthesia in both groups. The groups appeared to be too small to achieve statistical importance.

The similar pain control in both groups confirmed previous investigations [9–12]. The different temperature changes observed in the infrared photos present us with

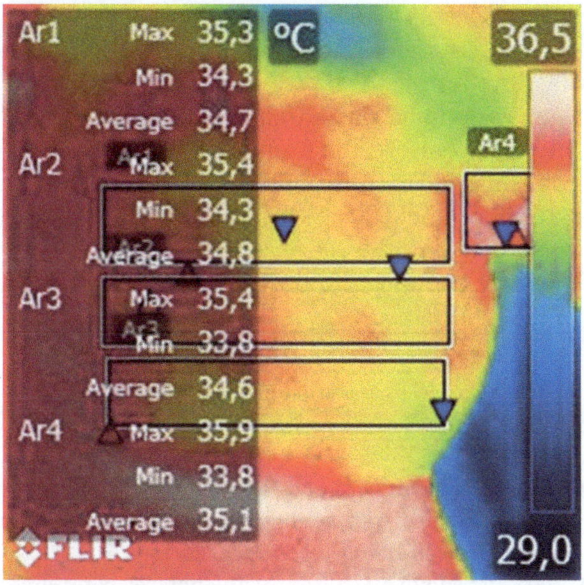

Figure 15.6. Infrared photo taken before analgesia in the one-shot group.

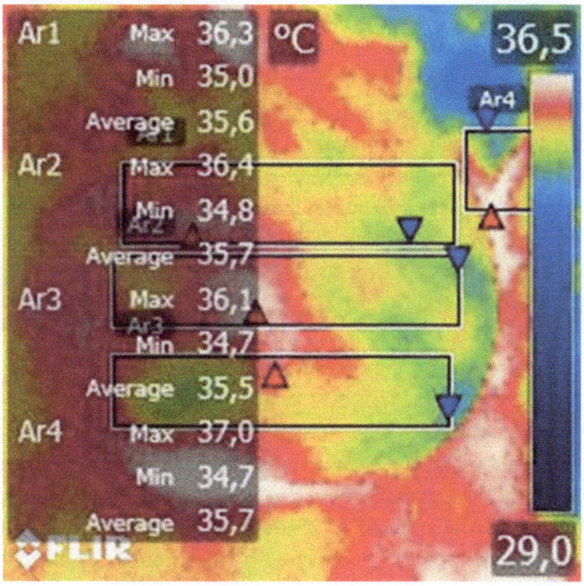

Figure 15.7. Infrared photo 20 min after TPVB, in the one-shot group.

a challenge. We assume that increase of temperature in the middle and lower regions rather than in upper region is related to the easier caudal spread of anaesthetic in the round fascia area, which has been mentioned previously [13–15]. The relatively higher number of patients with temperature increases in the M group in our opinion may prove that this technique creates the faster onset of the nerve block.

The results give no answer as to which technique is more effective as an analgesia method for elective breast surgery but may support the theory that the multi-shot method provides faster effects and allows earlier surgery onset. In the reality of operating room organization and the search for cost-effectiveness without compromising patient safety and comfort, the multi-shot technique can be recommended. The results are promising and in our opinion prove that infrared imaging can be used in the evaluation of the efficacy of the TPVB in breast surgery and in experimental studies evaluating the range and efficacy of different kinds of nerve blocks. This study will be continued to obtain more reliable data.

References

[1] Karmarkar M K 2001 Thoracic paravertebral blockade *Anesthesiology* **95** 771–80

[2] Gilbert J and Hultman J 1989 Thoracic paravertebral block: a method of pain control *Acta Anaesth. Scand.* **33** 142–5

[3] Karmakar M K, Chui P T, Joynt G M and Ho A M 2001 Thoracic paravertebral block for management of pain associated with multiple fractures ribs in patients with concomitant lumbar spinal trauma *Regional Anesth. Pain Med.* **26** 169–73

[4] Lönnqvist P-A 2005 Pre-emptive analgesia with thoracic paravertebral blockade? *Br. J. Anaesth.* **95** 6

[5] Ferrandiz M, Aliaga L, Catala E and Villar-Landeira J M 1994 Thoracic paravertebral block in chronic postoperative pain *Regional Anesth.* **19** 221–2

[6] Wang J Y 2000 Post-thoracotomy epidural versus paravertebral analgesia *Br. J. Anaesth.* **84** 289–90

[7] Możański M, Rustecki B, Kalicki B and Jung A 2015 Thermal evaluation of paravertebral block for mastectomy in high risk patient: case report *J. Clin. Monit. Comput.* **29** 297–9

[8] Machura W, Rustecki B, Klimkiewicz J, Możański M, Jung A and Kalicki B 2015 Infrared evaluation of efficacy of thoracic paravertebral block—preliminary study *19th Congr. Polish Association of Thermology (20–22 March 2015, Zakopane)*

[9] Cheema S P S, Ilsley D, Richardson J and Sabanathan S 1995 A thermographic study of paravertebral analgesia *Anesthesia* **50** 118–21

[10] Moller J F, Nikolajsen L, Rodt S A, Ronning H and Carlsson P S 2007 Thoracic paravertebral block for breast cancer surgery: a randomized double-blind study *Anesth. Analgesia* **105** 1848–51

[11] Kairaluoma P M, Bachmann M S, Korpinen A K, Rosenberg P H and Pere P J 2004 Single injection paravertebral block before general anesthesia enhances analgesia after breast cancer surgery with and without associated lymph node biopsy *Anesth. Analgesia* **99** 1837–43

[12] Naja Z M, El-Rejab M, Al-Tannir M A, Ziade F M, Tayara K, Younes F and Lonnqvist P A 2004 Thoracic paravertebral block: influence of the number of injections *Regional Anesth Pain Med.* **29** 5

[13] Cheema S P S, ILsley D, Richardson J and Sabanathan S 1995 A thermografic study of paravertebral analgesia *Anesthesia* **50** 118–21

[14] Marhofer D, Marhofer P, Kettner S C, Fleischmann E, Prayer D, Schernthaner M, Lackner E, Wilschke H, Schwetz P and Zeitlinger M 2013 Magnetic resonance imaging analysis of spread of local anesthetic solution after ultrasound-guided local thoracic paravertebral blockade *J. Am. Soc. Anesthesiologists* **118** 1106–12

[15] Richardson J, Jones J and Atkinson R 1998 The effect of thoracic paravertebral blockade on intercostal somatosensory evoked potentials *Anesth. Analgesia* **87** 373–6

Chapter 16

The sensitivity of infrared imaging for diagnosing Raynaud's phenomenon is dependent on the method of temperature extraction from thermal images*

16.1 Introduction

Raynaud's phenomenon is characterized by colour changes of the fingers and, occasionally, of the toes. Pallor (or white fingers) is caused by arterial vasoconstriction, cyanosis (or blue fingers) is due to venous congestion and rubor (or redness of fingers) is the result of reactive hyperemia. White fingers are often accompanied by a low skin temperature and thermal imaging was already used in the 1970s for the diagnosis of Raynaud's phenomenon [1–3].

Immersion of hands in water of 20 °C is a well-accepted cold challenge test for the thermographic diagnosis of Raynaud's phenomenon [4]. However, a standard for the evaluation of temperature changes has not yet been established. Francis Ring proposed a thermal index by combining the temperature gradients from the dorsum to the fingers prior to and after the cold challenge [5]. Others have determined the gradient of single fingers [6] or used the slope of the rewarming curve [7, 8].

16.2 Methods

Three methods of evaluation of temperature readings from thermal images were compared in the hands of 26 subjects after thermal images were recorded in the following way. After acclimatization for 15 min to a room temperature of 24 °C, the hands were positioned on a table and images in the dorsal view for both hands were recorded. Then the hands, covered with plastic gloves, were fully immersed for 1 min

*Partly reproduced from Ammer K 2008 *Thermol. Int.* **18** 81–8.

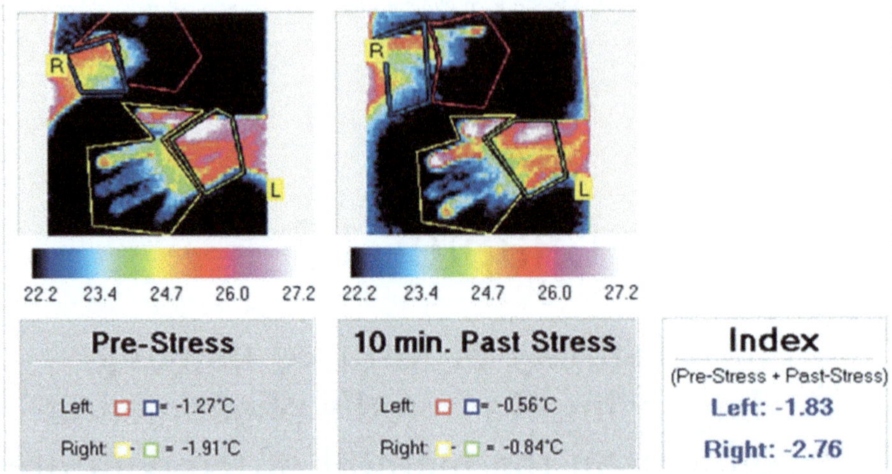

Figure 16.1. Example of the cold stress tool of CTHERM that generates the thermal index.

in water of 20 °C. Immediately after taking off the gloves and after intervals of 10 and 20 min three thermal images were captured.

The cold stress test tool of the software package C-THERM was used for the calculation of Ring's thermal index. Ring originally [9] excluded the thumb from the ROI due to the fact that the thumb is rarely affected by Raynaud's phenomenon, which was confirmed by the study in [10]. However, we included all of the fingers in the distal measurement area (figure 16.1).

Briefly, the thermal index was calculated in the following way. In the image prior to the cold challenge the distal ROI (ROI 1) including the thumb and all of the long fingers was defined by the statistics tool of CTHERM. Next ROI 2 was defined from the wrist to the metacarpal (MCP) joints. The programme automatically calculates the mean temperatures of the measurement fields. This procedure was repeated for the images 10 and 20 min after the cold challenge. Finally, two images of interest were imported into the cold stress tool of CTHERM, where the temperature difference between the distal and proximal ROIs is automatically calculated and the thermal index is generated by summing up the temperature differences in the earlier and the later image.

Alternatively, areas over single fingers were defined and gradients of single fingers were calculated by subtracting the mean temperature of the dorsum from the mean temperature of the finger areas (FG1 = finger gradient 1) (figure 16.2). Combining the mean FG1 prior to and after the cold challenge resulted in a thermal index area (TI_a).

The temperature gradients for single fingers were determined in the following way (figure 16.3). Spot temperatures were measured on the tip and over the middle of the MCP bone of each finger. The gradients were calculated by subtracting the MCP temperature from the temperature of the fingertip (FG2 = finger gradient 2). The mean values of the temperature gradients of all fingers of the right and the left hand were calculated.

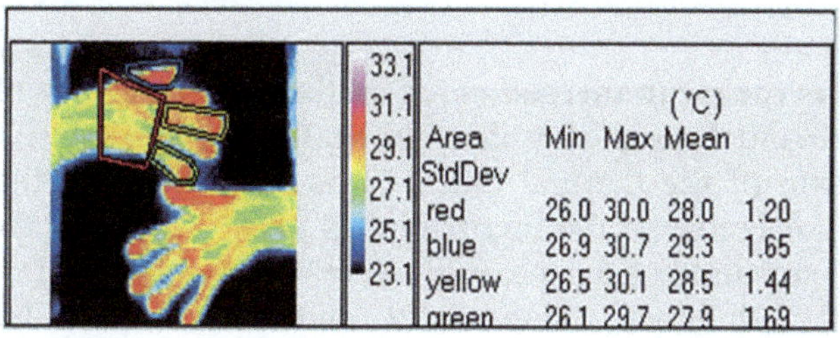

Figure 16.2. Combination of a measurement area over the dorsal hand with a measurement area over each finger.

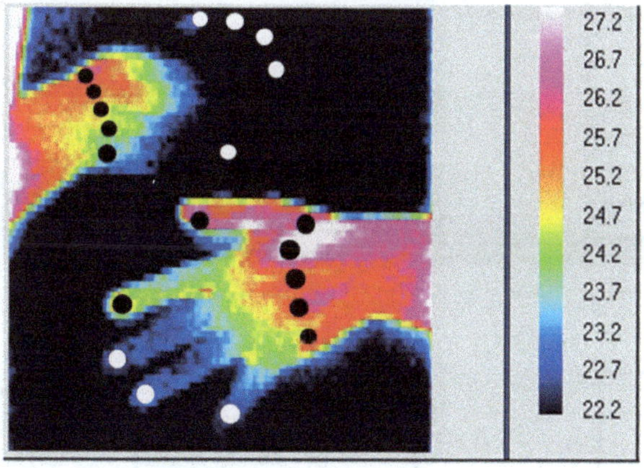

Mean thermal gradient (mTG)
mTG left: –2.22
mTG right: –2.76

	Before Stress									
	R1	R2	R3	R4	R5	L1	L2	L3	L4	L5
Finger tip	22.7	22.0	22.0	22.0	22.0	26.4	25.0	22.6	22.9	22.6
Metacarpal	25.7	25.4	25.1	24.3	24.0	28.0	25.4	25.5	26.0	25.7
Gradient	–3.0	–3.4	–3.1	–2.3	–2.0	–1.6	–0.4	–2.9	–3.1	–3.1

Figure 16.3. Definition of temperature gradients of single fingers.

An alternative thermal index gradient (TI_g) was calculated by summing up the mean temperature gradients of the fingers in the images of interest, i.e. the comparison of the image prior to the cold challenge with the image 10 or 20 min after the cold challenge.

16.3 Statistical evaluation

Using the software package SPSS 10, the three thermal indices were statistically analysed using non-parametric tests. The level for significant differences was set to two-tailed $p = 0.05$. The reliability coefficient α and the average interclass correlation were also calculated.

Diagnosis of Raynaud's phenomenon was based on a thermal index greater than –4.00 [5]. The frequency of the occurrence of Raynaud's phenomenon from the different methods was compared using the chi-square test.

16.4 Results

Figure 16.4 shows the mean thermal index on the right hand side obtained from all three methods 10 and 20 min after the cold challenge.

The comparison of the thermal index 10 and 20 min after the cold challenge obtained a mean decrease of the thermal index of 0.32 ± 1.0 at the later measurement. The absolute values of the mean TI_a were 0.93 to 1.28 greater than the related thermal index. The differences between TI_g and the thermal index were 0.1 to 1.

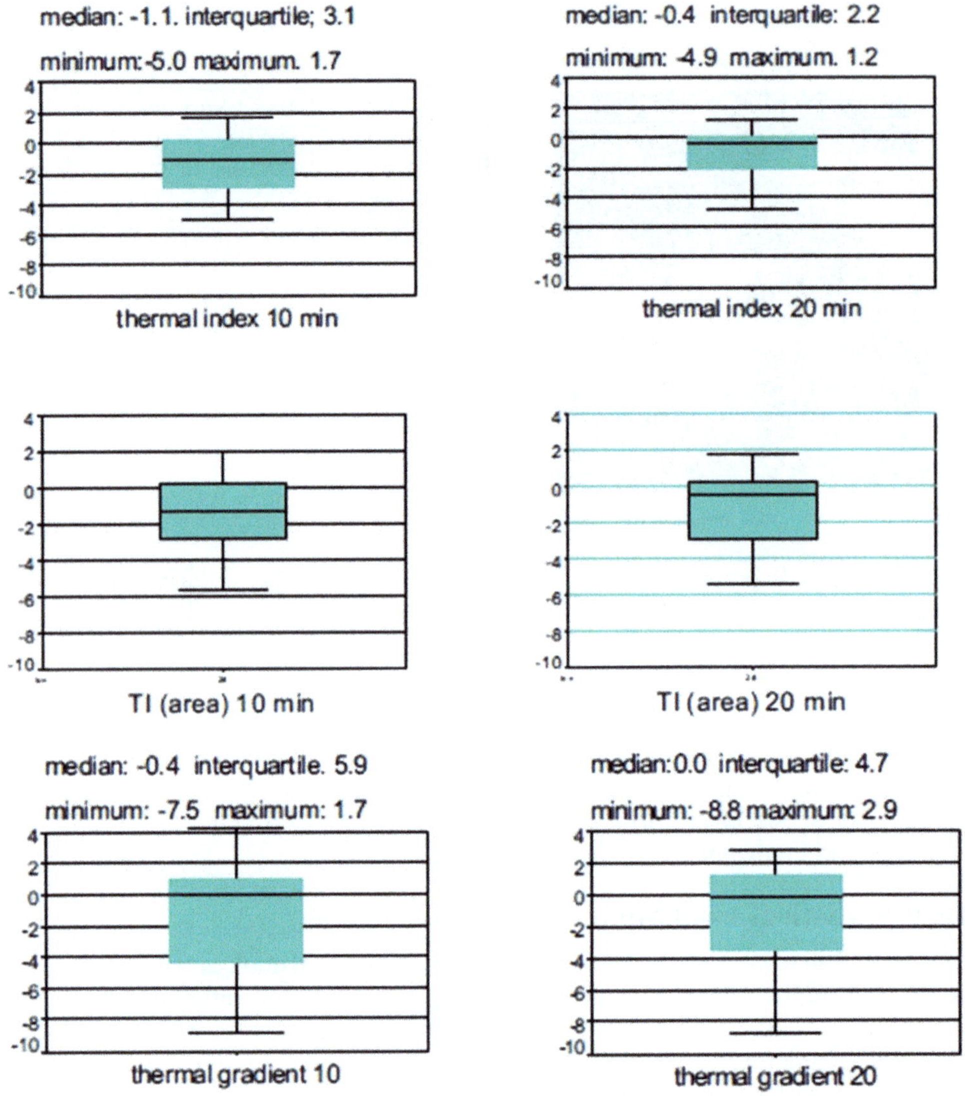

Figure 16.4. Mean thermal indices at the right hand side.

Table 16.1. Cases with Raynaud's phenomenon detected by different methods of evaluation.

Time after cold challenge	TI_g	TI_a	Thermal index
10 min	13 cases	10 cases	7 cases
20 min	9 cases	5 cases	3 cases

However, analysing all the thermal indices with non-parametric tests obtained no significant differences between the indices. The single measure interclass correlations revealed values between 0.75 and 0.95.

Using a threshold of –4.0 for a diagnostic thermal index, the highest number of cases with Raynaud's phenomenon were identified using TI_g, followed by TI_a and then the C-THERM derived thermal index (table 16.1).

A high correlation was found between the thermal index determined by the dedicated tool of the software package C-THERM and an alternatively calculated thermal index based on the temperature gradient of single fingers and comparing measurement areas over the hand and over single fingers, respectively. However, the thermal index derived from the temperature gradients of single fingers may be more sensitive for diagnosis than the other two thermal indices.

16.5 Discussion

In both studies, smaller measurement areas resulted in a higher diagnostic sensitivity than larger ROIs. This might be caused by the higher accuracy of infrared based temperature measurements from small areas taken from objects with a curved surface as the loss of radiation beyond a viewing angle of 45° may become critical [11, 12].

However, precision is higher when the measurement areas cover the total field of interest and are not just placed somewhere within the ROI. Following the outline of the fingers in the thermal images revealed a high intra- and inter-reader repeatability of temperature readings, even in images with poor thermal contrast [12]. An hourglass shaped ROI which aligned much better to the outline of the anterior knee than a circular or rectangular measurement area also resulted in high repeatability of temperature measures [13].

As the accuracy and precision of infrared based temperature measurements confer a different weight and importance for a diagnostic test and for an outcome measure [14], appropriate definition of measurement area may vary due to the intended utility of the thermal imaging.

16.6 Conclusion

Different methods of evaluation lead to different sensitivities of thermal imaging. More cases of Raynaud's phenomenon were diagnosed with smaller measurement areas than with large ROIs.

References

[1] Thiers H, Schmitt M and Fayolle J 1970 Donnees thermographiques dans les syndromes de Raynaud. Premiers resultats lyonnais *Bull. Soc. Fr. Dermatol. Syphiligr.* **77** 462–4

[2] Chucker F, Fowler R, Motomiya T and Hurley W 1971 Transients in Raynaud's disease measured by thermography: a preliminary report *Andrology* **22** 580–93

[3] Brachtel R and Schramm P 1978 Telethermography and infrared thermometry in the diagnosis of Raynaud-like symptoms *Med. Welt.* **29** 588–94

[4] Ring E F J *et al* 1988 Raynaud's phenomenon: assessment by thermography *Thermology* **3** 69–73

[5] Ring E F J 1980 A thermographic index for the assessment of ischemia *Acta Thermographica* **5** 35–8

[6] Ammer K 1996 Diagnosis of Raynaud's phenomenon by thermography *Skin Res. Technol.* **2** 182–5

[7] Boesinger P and Geser H M 1999 A thermodynamic model for thermographic analysis of tissue perfusion and its regulation *Thermology* **3** 191–8

[8] Merla A, Di Donato L, Di Luzio S and Luca Romani G 2002 Quantifying the relevance and stage of disease with the tau image technique *IEEE Eng. Med. Biol.* **21** 86–92

[9] Chikura B, Moore T L, Manning J B, Vail A and Herrick A L 2008 Sparing of the thumb in Raynaud's phenomenon *Rheumatology* **47** 219–21

[10] Clark J A 1976 Effects of surface emissivity and viewing angle errors in thermography *Acta Thermographica* **1** 138–41

[11] Ammer K 2003 Need for standardisation of measurements in thermal imaging *Thermography and Lasers in Medicine* ed B Wiecek (Lodz: Akademickie Centrum Graficzno-Marketigowe Lodart SA) pp 13–18

[12] Melnizky P, Schartelmüller T and Ammer K 1997 Prüfung der intra- und indinterindividuellen Verläßlichkeit der Auswertung von Infrarot-Thermogrammen *Eur. J. Thermol.* **7** 224–7

[13] Ammer K, Ring E F J, Plassmann P and Jones B F 2002 Rationale for standardised capture and analysis of infrared thermal images (*Proc. European Medical and Biological Engineering Conf. Part II*) ed H Hutten and P Krösel (Graz: IFMBE) pp 1608–9

[14] Ammer K 2006 Thermal imaging as an outcome measure *Thermol. Int.* **16** 125

Chapter 17

Nerve entrapment and skin temperature of the human hand

17.1 Carpal tunnel syndrome and thoracic outlet syndrome

Carpal tunnel syndrome (CTS) and the mild form of thoracic outlet syndrome (TOS) are frequently seen nerve entrapments. Both disorders are often associated with changes of the skin temperature of the human hand.

Skin temperature is maintained by the perfusion of skin vessels under the control of the sympathetic nervous system. High sympathetic activity caused by reasons other than thermoregulation leads to vasoconstriction, but a total loss of sympathetic control is followed by an increase in heat emission from the skin.

Entrapments of peripheral nerves result in neuropraxia or in structural changes of nerve fibres. This pathology leads to disturbed blood circulation within the nerve which is followed by pain and activation of the sympathetic nervous system.

Most nerve entrapment syndromes can be detected by thermal imaging with cool areas of skin temperature localized in the sensory distribution areas of the affected nerves (figure 17.1). In CTS severe compression of the median nerve may lead to a total loss of the autonomic control and an increase of the skin temperature of the first three fingers (figure 17.2).

Thermal changes of the skin may sometimes only be observed after provocation tests as in TOS where arm raising causes pressure on the nerve. In most patients with the mild form of TOS the lower portion of the brachial plexus is affected, resulting in a cold little finger (figure 17.3). Combinations of CTS and TOS may be found in some patients (figure 17.4). In most of these cases the thermal pattern of TOS predominates the temperature changes of CTS.

In either form of nerve entrapment on the arm, diagnostic evidence is achieved by a temperature difference in the sensory distribution areas of the affected nerves greater than 0.5 °C.

doi:10.1088/978-0-7503-1143-4ch17

17.2 Evaluation of thoracic outlet syndrome

In images from patients with suspected TOS, the ROIs are placed on the index and the little finger. The outline of the measuring shape crosses the index (little finger) at the inter-digital fold, follows the outline of the finger and returns to the starting point.

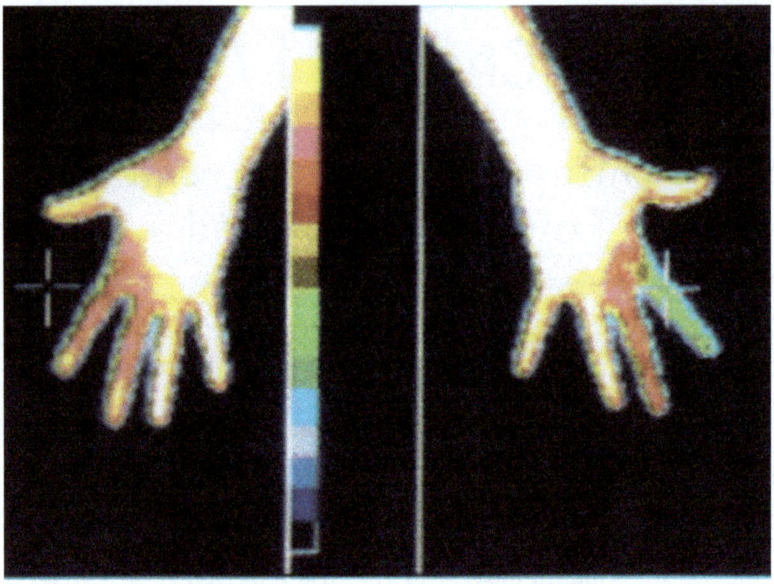

Figure 17.1. 41-year-old female patient with delayed nerve conduction velocity of the sensory nerve fibres of both median nerves presenting with low skin temperature of the index and middle finger bilaterally.

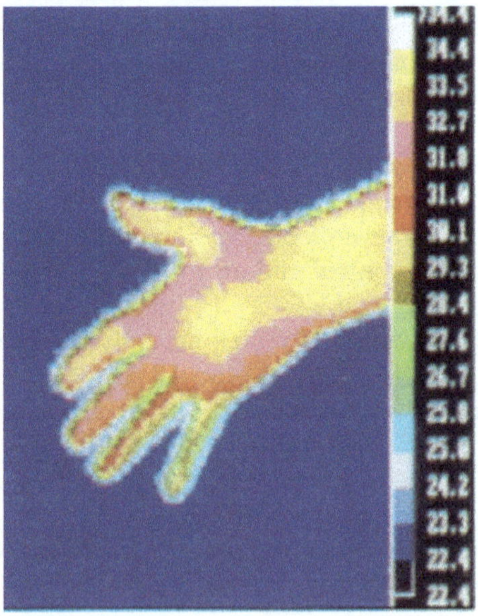

Figure 17.2. 76-year-old male patient four weeks after surgical treatment of severe CTS (distal latency prior to operation 6.7 ms) presenting with hyperthermia of the first three fingers.

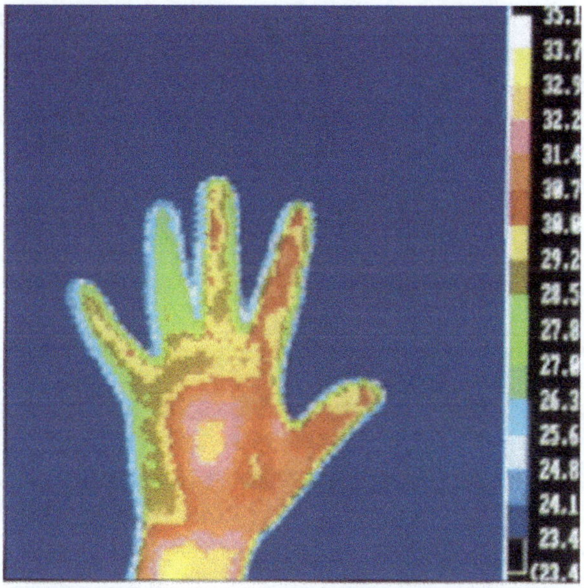

Figure 17.3. 41-year-old female patient with normal electrophysiological findings and symptoms of a mild form of TOS on the right-hand side presenting with a cold fourth and fifth finger during the hyperabduction test.

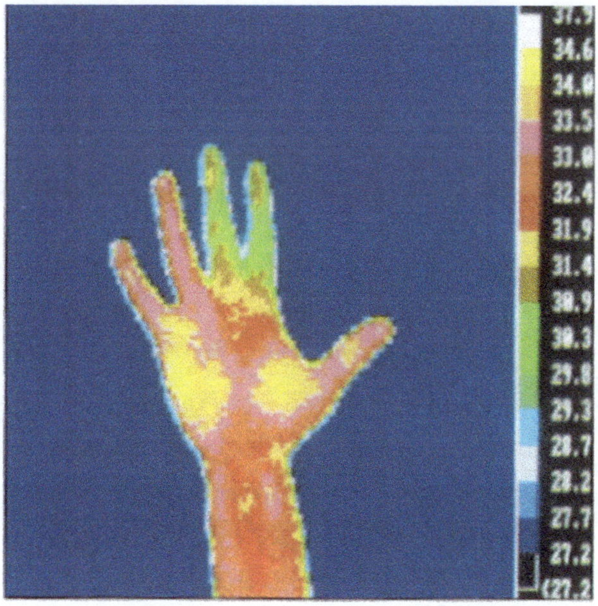

Figure 17.4. 44-year-old male patient with mild CTS (distal latency 4.5 ms) and clinical symptoms of a mild form of TOS on the right-hand side presenting with a cold second and third finger during the hyperabduction test.

Such ROIs must be generated for each image of thoracic outlet series (position $1a_1$: right palm, $1a_2$: left palm, 1b: both palms placed on a table; position 2: hands up, 2_1: right hand, 2_2: left hand; position 3: hyperabduction, 3_1: right hand, 3_2: left hand; position 4: modified Adson test, 4_1: right hand, 4_2: left hand). Figure 17.5 shows a series of thermograms recorded in a patient with suspected TOS.

The difference in mean temperature of the index finger and the little finger is less than 0.5 °C in healthy subjects, differences of 0.5 °C or more are regarded

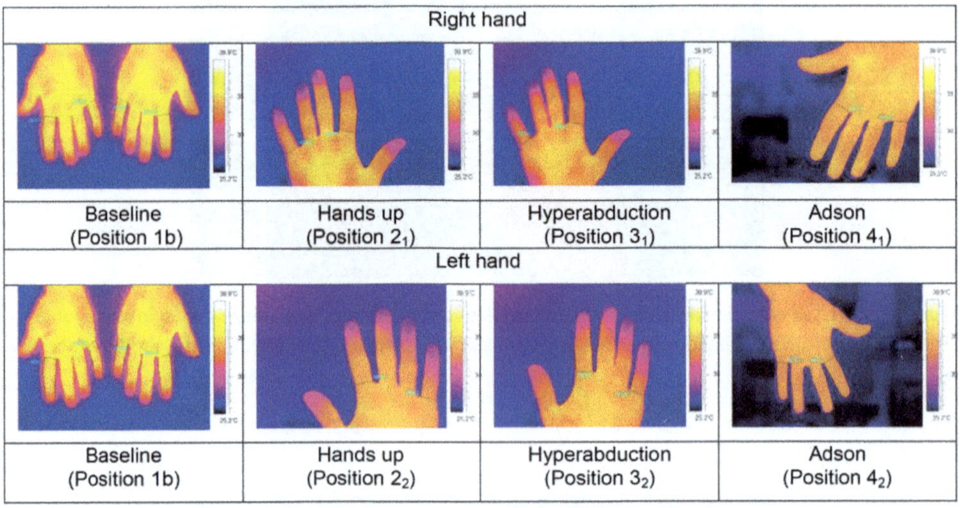

Figure 17.5. Thermal images of a patient with bilateral 'probable' TOS

Table 17.1.

	Right hand			
	Baseline (°C)	Hands up (°C)	Hyperabduction (°C)	Adson (°C)
Index finger	34.4	32.5	32.4	33.6
Little finger	34.1	31.5	31.3	33.2
Temperature difference	0.31	**0.99**	**1.72**	0.37
	Left hand			
	Baseline (°C)	Hands up (°C)	Hyperabduction (°C)	Adson (°C)
Index finger	34.4	32.3	32.5	33.6
Little finger	34.2	31.1	31.2	33.2
Temperature difference	0.24	**1.22**	**1.24**	0.35

as abnormal. Based on such temperature differences the following classification was made:

- an abnormal temperature difference in one position was named 'possible TOS',
- abnormal findings in two positions was regarded as 'probable TOS' and
- abnormal temperature readings in three or four arm positions was classified as 'definite TOS'.

In addition, TOS cases were labelled with 'index' or 'little finger' with respect to the colder finger. Table 17.1 shows the temperature findings of a patient with bilateral 'probable TOS'.

In cases of suspected CTS the same ROIs (index and little finger) should be used and applied to the image of the dorsal hands.

Chapter 18

Imaging assessments of patients with suspected systemic sclerosis and associated inflammatory lung disease

18.1 Description

Patients with SSc, also known as scleroderma, experience significant morbidity and mortality [1, 2]. Hallmarks of SSc include inflammation, tissue fibrosis, production of certain antibodies and impaired microvascular perfusion. An early diagnosis helps to implement the most appropriate therapy for each patient and thus improve quality of life and survival. Some patients can also have linked ILD and this also needs careful assessment to stage the severity of disease.

18.2 Clinical presentation

A 45-year-old man presented to his general practitioner with recent onset Raynaud's symptoms which were reported as worsening in frequency and severity of attacks. The patient had also noticed increasing breathlessness on mild exertion and significant fatigue over the last few months. The patient was referred to the Newcastle combined connective tissue disease ILD clinic for an expert opinion by a consultant rheumatologist (author BG) and a consultant in respiratory medicine (author IF).

18.3 Investigations and procedures, diagnostic findings

The patient underwent a full multi-system clinical assessment by a consultant rheumatologist specializing in connective tissue disease. An immunological screen was also performed. The imaging work up included standard microvascular imaging by author JA at the Microvascular Diagnostics measurement facility at Freeman Hospital with dynamic thermal imaging (giving a thermoregulatory microcirculation assessment) and nail fold capillaroscopy (giving a nutritional microcirculation assessment) [3]. A HRCT scan of the chest was also performed.

doi:10.1088/978-0-7503-1143-4ch18

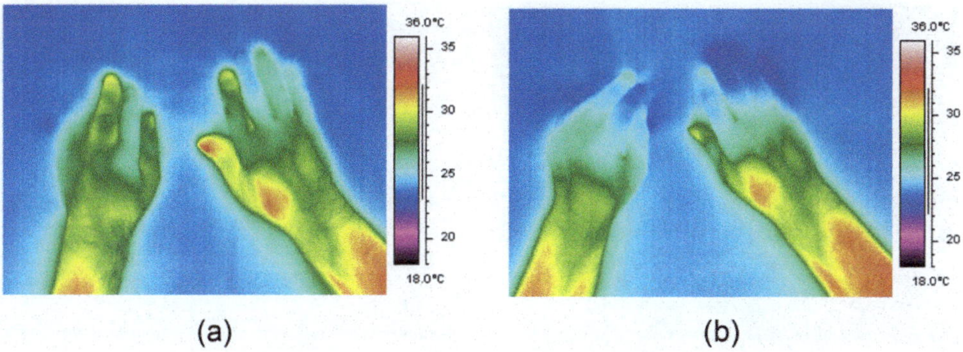

Figure 18.1. (*a*) Baseline thermal image showing clear thermal asymmetry and unevenness at the fingers. (*b*) 10 min after the mild cold challenge most fingers remained cold. The summed thermal gradients would be consistent with Raynaud's. The patchy thermal presentation at rest and clear thermal asymmetry at the thumbs could point to a secondary Raynaud's condition. An area of relative warmth can also be seen at the base of the right thumb which can be an indication of local joint inflammation.

For the microvascular imaging the patient followed the pre-imaging protocol instructions which included avoiding any smoking, caffeinated substances and talc/creams on the skin of the hands on the day of their test. They arrived at the hospital and were acclimatized for 30 min in the waiting room and then moved into the temperature and humidity controlled room for imaging at the normothermic setting (23.5 °C, 40–50% relative humidity). The standard thermography testing included a 10 min baseline, a 1 min mild cold challenge of the hands in a water bucket at 20 °C (the patient wore light surgical gloves whilst the hands were immersed), followed by a period of 10 min to allow and monitor any re-warming of the fingers with a thermal camera (FLIR Systems SC300) [4]. The summed thermal gradients of the fingers, from baseline plus 10 min following the mild cold challenge, were evaluated to assess any prolonged vasospasm. The thermal unevenness across the fingers and any asymmetry between the hands were assessed (figure 18.1). After the thermography the patient underwent nail fold capillaroscopy with an assessment of capillary loop morphology using a purpose built microscope with a wide field view (×100 lens, KK Technology). A total of six fingers (right and left index, middle and ring fingers) were studied with capillaroscopy to look for features of connective tissue disease related microangiopathy which included loop dilatation, avascular fields, extravasation and angiogenesis [5] (figure 18.2).

18.4 Brief discussion and conclusion

Thermal imaging in combination with nail fold capillaroscopy has shown evidence for Raynaud's secondary to a connective tissue disease in the scleroderma spectrum pattern. These are powerful tests when used in combination. Although auscultation of the chest was normal, in addition, the HRCT chest scan showed evidence of ILD (figure 18.3). The immunological tests (anti-Scl-70 antibody) were also abnormal in this patient. The patient also had puffy fingers and mild sclerodactyly. This patient had early definite SSc, as defined by the 2013 classification criteria for SSc [6]. This patient's disease was rapidly progressive.

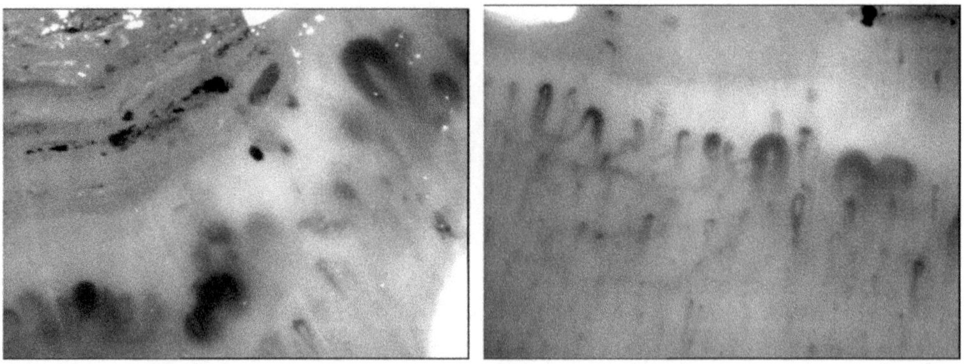

Figure 18.2. Example of abnormal capillaroscopy images from two fingers. There are clear abnormalities, including local dilatation to the grade of giant loop, clear avascular regions, spots of extravasation and architectural disorganization. These features of microangiopathy were seen in most fingers studied and would be consistent with a scleroderma spectrum pattern. It is noted that the finger site is chosen as it is accessible and a place where the capillaries usually lie parallel to the skin surface allowing their full structure to be observed with the microscope. Microangiopathy at the nail fold may indicate microangiopathy in the vital organs of the body.

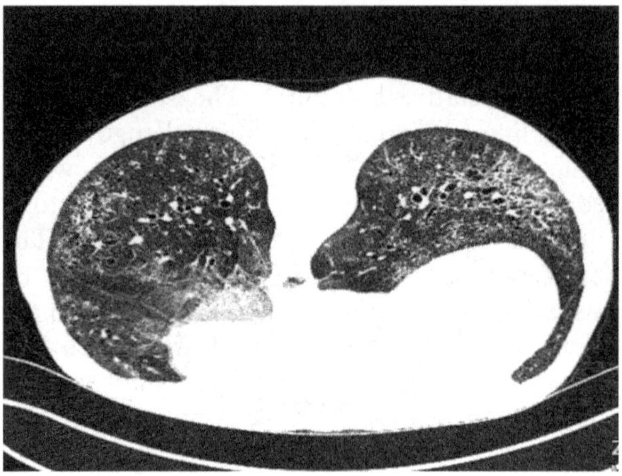

Figure 18.3. HRCT chest scan showing clear regions attributed to lung tissue fibrosis and also inflammation bilaterally for a patient with established ILD.

All tests are essential pieces of the diagnostic jigsaw from which the expert physician can determine the correct diagnosis and determine appropriate treatment pathways.

References

[1] Steen V D and Medsger T A 2007 Changes in causes of death in systemic sclerosis *Ann. Rheumatic Diseases* **66** 940–4

[2] Cutolo M, Sulli A and Smith V 2010 Assessing microvascular changes in systemic sclerosis diagnosis and management *Nat. Rev. Rheumatol.* **6** 578–87

[3] Allen J and Howell K J 2014 Clinical microvascular imaging: techniques and opportunities for clinical physiological measurements *Physiol. Meas.* **35** R91–141
[4] Kumar N, Allen J, Murray A and Griffiths B 2006 The assessment of single dose Sildenafil Citrate (Viagra) in the treatment of Raynaud's phenomenon in patients with systemic sclerosis *J. Rheumatol.* **33** 1918–19
[5] Cutolo M 2010 *Atlas of Capillaroscopy in Rheumatic Diseases* (Amsterdam: Elsevier)
[6] van den Hoogen F *et al* 2013 Classification criteria for systemic sclerosis: an American College of Rheumatology/European League Against Rheumatism collaborative initiative *Arthritis Rheumatol.* **65** 2737–47

Chapter 19

The use of infrared thermography to differentiate 'cold intolerance' from 'true Raynaud's phenomenon' in the context of fibromyalgia

19.1 Case history

Raynauds phenomenon has been described since its first identification in 1862 [1–3]. A 43-year-old woman presented to the Rheumatology department with typical symptoms of FMS including widespread hyperalgesia, low mood, un-refreshing sleep and intolerance to bright light and loud noises. She also described increased sensitivity to cold with pain, numbness and white/blue discolouration of the digits of her hands and feet in response to cold exposure (suggestive of RP).

On examination, she had widespread myofascial tenderness with pain stimulated by palpation over 16 of the 18 fibromyalgia tender points [4]. There were no stigmata of connective tissue disease, inflammatory arthritis or other systemic illness.

Blood tests demonstrated unremarkable full blood count, renal and liver function tests, calcium profile, plasma viscosity and C reactive protein. Anti-tissue transglutaminate antibodies were within the normal range (NR). Immunofluorescence on human epithelial (HEp2) cells revealed non-specific anti-nuclear antibody staining of doubtful significance. ELISA studies to identify antibody specificity to extractable nuclear antigens and DNA-binding were negative. The thyroid stimulating hormone level was borderline raised at 5.27 mIU L^{-1} (NR 0.3–5.0 mIU L^{-1}) with markedly raised anti-thyroid peroxidase antibodies of 837 IU mL^{-1} (NR $<$ 101 IU mL^{-1}) suggestive of early autoimmune hypothyroidism, although she was clinically and biochemically euthyroid with a normal free T4 of 13.6 pmol L^{-1} (12.0–22.0 pmol L^{-1}).

The patient underwent a standardized cold stress test to allow dynamic assessment of digital microvascular function. Following 20 min acclimatization (at 23 °C +/−0.5 °C), thermographic images were taken of the dorsum of the hands

doi:10.1088/978-0-7503-1143-4ch19

(Thermovision Camera, FLIR systems, Danderyd, Sweden). Her hands were then submerged (in polythene gloves to avoid evaporative cooling) to the level of the radio-carpal joint into a water bath cooled to 20 °C (+/−0.1 °C) for 60 s. A second thermal image of the dorsum of the hands was captured 10 min after the cold challenge. All images were processed using CTHERM software (version 2.3, University of Glamorgan). Regions of interest encompassing the digits and dorsum of the hand were prepared and the mean temperature recorded (see figure 19.1). The thermal gradient (TG, temperature of digits minus dorsum) at the baseline was +0.4 and +0.2 for the right and left hand, respectively (suggesting normal basal microvascular tone within the digital arteriovenous anastomoses). The TG following the cold challenge was +0.8 and +0.4 for the right and left hand, respectively, which would not support an exaggerated response to cold exposure or delayed re-warming (figure 19.1).

NC was performed at the index, middle and ring fingers of each hand using a pillar mounted 1.3 mega-pixel camera (PL-A742, PixeLINK) at a magnification of ×200. The NC images did not reveal any structural morphological microvascular abnormalities at the nailfold (figure 19.2)

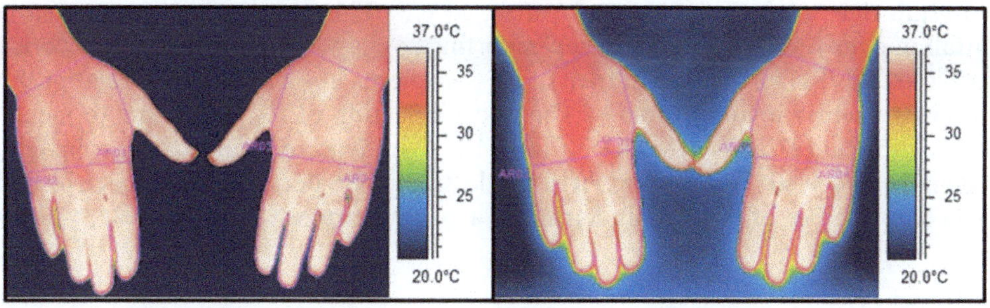

Figure 19.1. Thermographic assessment of the dorsum of the hands at the baseline and post-cold-challenge. The digital and dorsal regions of interest are included on the thermographic images taken at baseline (left) and 10 min post cold challenge (right).

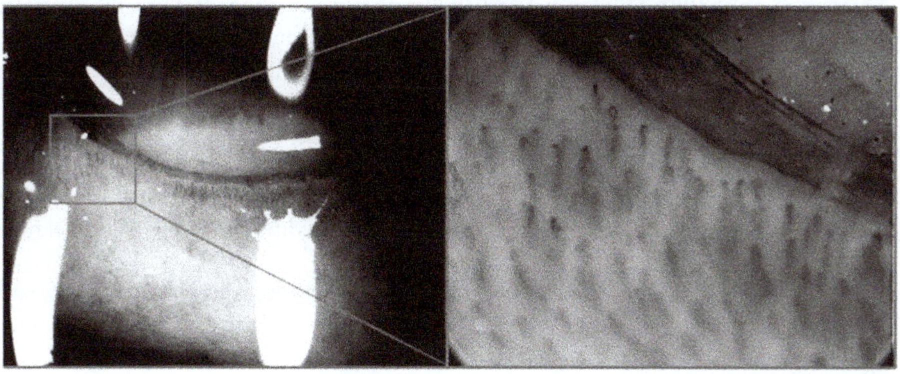

Figure 19.2. NC images obtained from the right middle finger. The image on the left is taken at 50× magnification, whereas the image on the right is taken at 200× magnification. The nailfold capillaries are of uniform size, length and density with no evidence of significant abnormalities such as tortuous/dilated vessels or microhaemorrhages.

On the basis of the clinical history, examination findings, blood tests and microvascular imaging studies, a diagnosis of fibromyalgia was made and it was considered that her RP-like symptoms were more suggestive of 'cold intolerance', rather than 'true RP'.

19.2 Discussion

A high prevalence of RP symptoms (18.2–53.3%) has been observed in FMS [5–8]. Furthermore, a small number of studies have identified objective evidence of peripheral microvascular dysfunction in FMS, although these studies were generally small and often identified a poor relationship between RP symptoms and objective evidence of microvascular compromise [8–12]. FMS is a poorly understood disorder in which central sensitization to a number of external stimuli occurs; namely nociception but also light, sound and temperature. The absence of structural or functional microvascular disturbance on objective assessment (using NC and IRT) in the present case would suggest the RP-like symptoms were more representative of 'cold intolerance' rather than the excessive digital microvascular response to cold exposure that might be associated with true RP. This case highlights a potential pitfall in over-reliance on patient self-reporting to diagnose RP. Additional work is required to establish the true burden of RP symptoms in FMS and their relationship to microvascular imaging studies. The re-classification of RP-symptoms to include 'cold intolerance' and 'true RP', aided by non-invasive microvascular imaging techniques such as IRT, might help guide treatment decisions, particularly with respect to the use of potentially harmful vasoactive drugs.

References

[1] Wigley F M 2002 Clinical practice. Raynaud's phenomen *New Engl. J. Med.* **347** 1001–8

[2] Raynaud M 1862 De l'asphyxie locale et de la gangene symetrique des extremites *MD Thesis* Faculte de Medicine de Paris

[3] Brennan P *et al* 1993 Validity and reliability of three methods used in the diagnosis of Raynaud's phenomenon. The UK Scleroderma Study Group *Br. J. Rheumatol.* **32** 357–61

[4] Wolfe F *et al* 1990 The American College of Rheumatology 1990 criteria for the classification of fibromyalgia. Report of the multicenter criteria committee *Arthritis Rheumatol.* **33** 160–72

[5] Wolfe F *et al* 2009 Fibromyalgia, systemic lupus erythematosus (SLE), and evaluation of SLE activity *J. Rheumatol.* **36** 82–8

[6] Vaeroy H, Helle R, Forre O, Kass E and Terenius L 1988 Elevated CSF levels of substance P and high incidence of Raynaud phenomenon in patients with fibromyalgia: new features for diagnosis *Pain* **32** 21–26

[7] Dinerman H, Goldenberg D L and Felson D T 1986 A prospective evaluation of 118 patients with the fibromyalgia syndrome: prevalence of Raynaud's phenomenon, sicca symptoms, ANA, low complement, and Ig deposition at the dermal-epidermal junction *J. Rheumatol.* **13** 368–73

[8] Bennett R M *et al* 1991 Symptoms of Raynaud's syndrome in patients with fibromyalgia. A study utilizing the Nielsen test, digital photoplethysmography, and measurements of platelet alpha 2-adrenergic recepto *Arthritis Rheumatol.* **34** 264–9

[9] Morf S *et al* 2005 Microcirculation abnormalities in patients with fibromyalgia—measured by capillary microscopy and laser fluxmetry *Arthritis Res. Ther.* **7** R209–16

[10] Jeschonneck M, Grohmann G, Hein G and Sprott H 2000 Abnormal microcirculation and temperature in skin above tender points in patients with fibromyalgia *Rheumatology* **39** 917–21

[11] Frodin T, Bengtsson A and Skogh M 1988 Nail fold capillaroscopy findings in patients with primary fibromyalgia *Clin. Rheumatol.* **7** 384–8

[12] Lindh M, Johansson G, Hedberg M, Henning G B and Grimby G 1995 Muscle fiber characteristics, capillaries and enzymes in patients with fibromyalgia and controls *Scand. J. Rheumatol.* **24** 34–37

Chapter 20

Hand arm vibration syndrome documented by thermal imaging—a case report

20.1 Introduction

Hand arm vibration syndrome (HAVS) is an occupational condition that affects subjects exposed to vibrating tools at the workplace and needs an accurate quantitative and objective diagnostic test to aid clinicians in the judgment of the degree of injury and adequate treatment. An objective assessing method is needed to provide a permanent evidence record of the degree of injury. In the case of chronic or permanent injury an objective measure to specify an appropriate compensation is required.

A procedure involving medical thermal imaging (figure 20.1) was developed to monitor the hands exposed to an objective mechanical provocation test involving vertical vibration, for 2 min at 31.5 Hz and 36 m/s^2. This test was followed by a thermal provocation challenge (cold stress test (CST)) of the hand for a period of 1 min at 20 °C. Images were taken during the whole procedure. An image from a calibration source was taken before and after to ensure quality assurance.

20.2 Case history

A male subject of 52 years of age was a professional builder operating with vibration instruments (driller). He had a BMI of 24.1 and had right handed dominance. He was referred by a physician to perform this test being suspected of HAVS. The test was performed in an acclimatized lab with an environment temperature of 22 °C and a relative humidity of <50%. The subject was given a period of acclimatization of 15 min and the images were recorded with the subject seated in a chair. Both hands were positioned over a board in order to facilitate background contrast. The thermal camera used was a FLIR A40sc (with a resolution of 320 × 240, a precision of 80 mK and an accuracy of ±2% of the overall reading) with 45° lenses, mounted on a pillar stand pointing downwards at a 90° angle to the dorsum of the hand, which was at 1 m distance.

doi:10.1088/978-0-7503-1143-4ch20

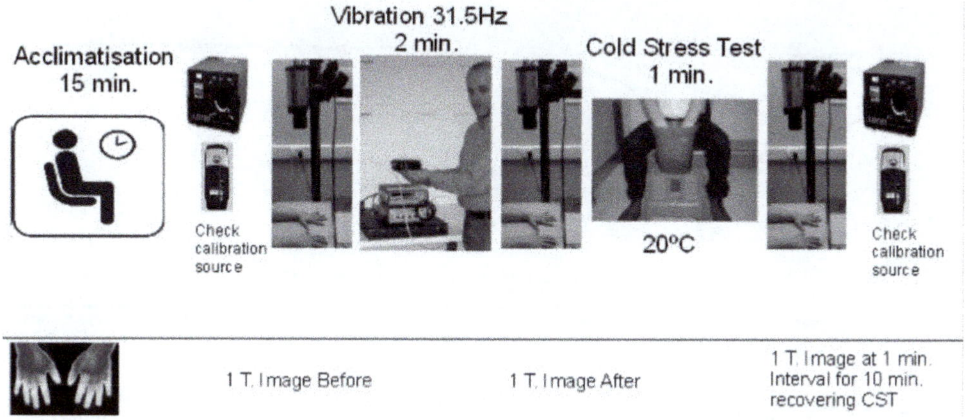

Figure 20.1. The HAVS provocation test procedure.

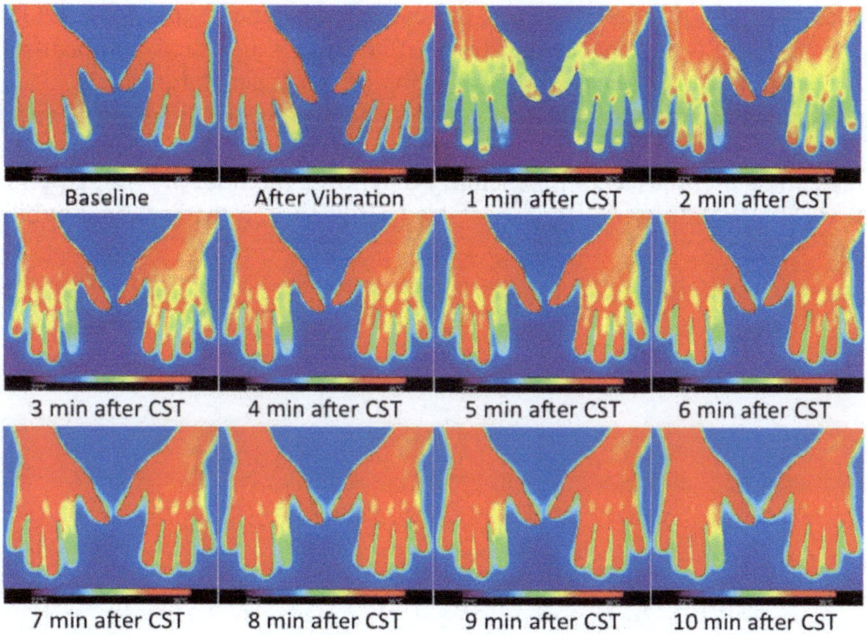

Figure 20.2. Thermal images taken during the whole procedure, from the period after acclimatization up to 10 min after the CST.

The mechanical provocation test consisted of an electrical device operating at a known frequency with a signal amplified and originated from a wave generator. This was held by the fingertips for 2 min. The thermal provocative stress consisted of a water bath at 20 °C, with the hands clothed in very thin plastic gloves and avoiding any contact. The hands were immersed in the water for 1 min.

The recorded thermal images are presented in figure 20.2, where it can be seen that the affected finger is the right index, the presence of a circulation defect can be seen and documented.

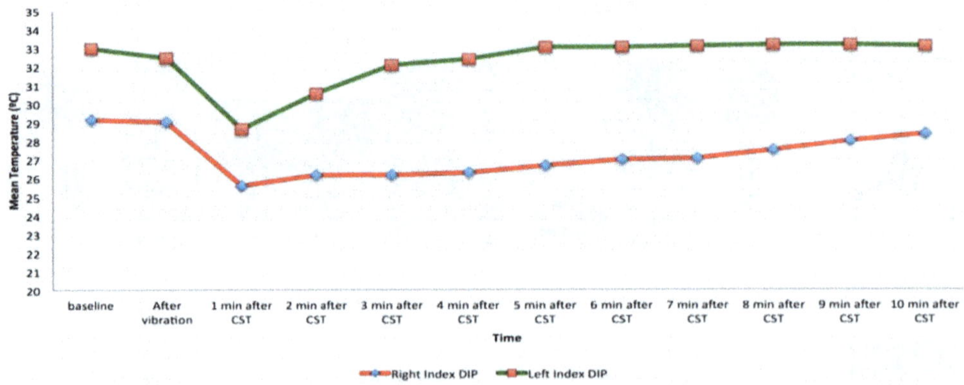

Figure 20.3. Comparison between the right and left DIP mean temperature during the provocation procedure.

Comparing the right index distal intra phalanx (DIP) mean temperature with the left index DIP mean temperature of the case study patient, using the CTHERM software package, it was shown that thermal imaging is an effective indicator of the severity of injury in the peripheral circulation of the finger (figure 20.3).

The proposed methodology is objective and repeatable, providing important physiological information of the evolutionary stage of HAVS. Medical thermal imaging can be useful as a complementary diagnostic method, providing permanent evidence of the condition in support of medical history in medico-legal liabilities.

IOP Publishing

Infrared Imaging
A casebook in clinical medicine
John Allen, Crispian Oates and David Talbot

Chapter 21

Thermal imaging and its potential for arterio-venous fistula function assessment

21.1 Description

AVFs, including synthetic grafts, are essential for the long-term treatment of end stage renal disease using haemodialysis [1, 2]. A fistula enables relatively risk-free and repeatable access to high volume blood flow rates. Vascular and clinical assessments of AVF function are therefore important to check for problems due to vascular steal or failure by occlusion. Vascular steal can affect digital blood flow and hence skin temperature. For example, if fistula flow is excessive then there can be blood flow steal from the hand on the side of the fistula which can result in ischaemia of the fingers. Objective non-invasive AVF assessment techniques available at Freeman Hospital include thermography [3, 4] and colour duplex ultrasound imaging [5].

21.2 Clinical presentation

Three adult patients were referred for thermography and AVF blood flow assessments. Clinically, one of the patients had a fistula which was well formed, the second showed evidence of vascular steal by discolouration of the fingers of the hand on the fistula side and the third had a fistula that was occluded and not viable, therefore, for renal dialysis. These three patients are an extract from our published paper on thermal imaging techniques for assessing renal fistulas [6].

21.3 Investigations and procedures, diagnostic findings

Imaging included standard microvascular imaging at the Microvascular Diagnostics measurement facility at Freeman Hospital, Newcastle upon Tyne, UK, with thermal imaging of the upper limbs/hands and also colour duplex ultrasound vascular imaging of patency and blood flow in the AVF (ATL HDI 5000 scanner fitted with a

doi:10.1088/978-0-7503-1143-4ch21

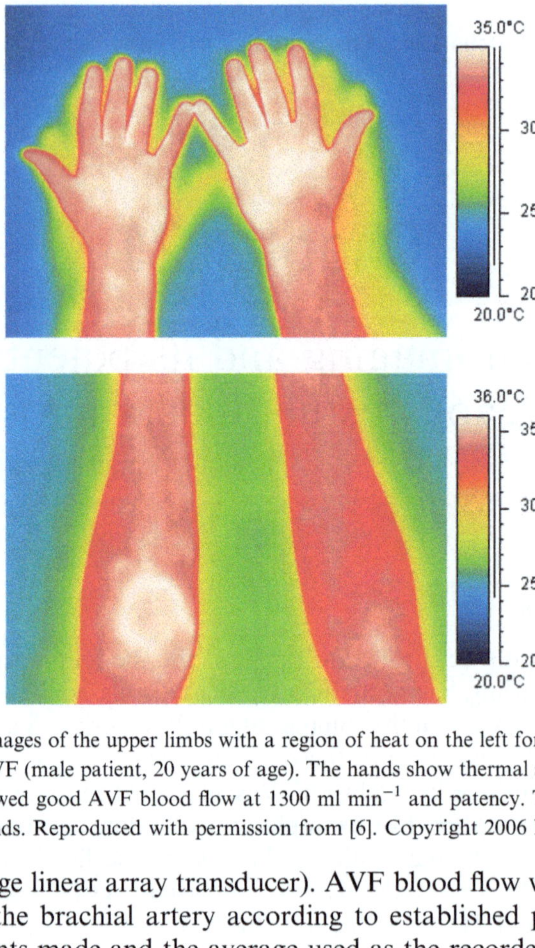

Figure 21.1. Thermal images of the upper limbs with a region of heat on the left forearm which is associated with the region of an AVF (male patient, 20 years of age). The hands show thermal symmetry. Colour duplex ultrasound imaging showed good AVF blood flow at 1300 ml min^{-1} and patency. There was no evidence of vascular steal at the hands. Reproduced with permission from [6]. Copyright 2006 IOP Publishing.

5.0–12.5 MHz range linear array transducer). AVF blood flow was estimated using measurements at the brachial artery according to established protocol with three repeat measurements made and the average used as the recorded blood flow.

For the thermal imaging the patient followed the pre-imaging protocol instructions which included avoiding any smoking, caffeinated substances and talc/creams on the skin of their hands on the day of their test. They arrived at the hospital and were acclimatized for 20 min in the waiting room and then moved into the temperature controlled room for imaging at the normothermic room setting (23.5 °C). The standard thermograpghy included imaging views of the upper arms, forearms and hands at rest using a thermal imaging camera (FLIR Systems SC300) [5]. Differences in hand temperature and maximum fistula/contra-lateral side regional temperatures were all determined using dedicated image processing software (FLIR ThermaCam Researcher, skin emissivity = 0.97) [6].

Thermal images are shown of the arms and hands in each of the three patient cases. Figure 21.1 shows a well performing AVF with a clear heat pattern around the fistula area on the forearm and no evidence of vascular steal from the hands. Figure 21.2(*a*) shows the case of vascular steal from the hand on the fistula side from excessive fistula flow and figure 21.2(*b*) shows the case of a likely occluded fistula. The duplex ultrasound measurements backed up these findings. Figure 21.3 shows a

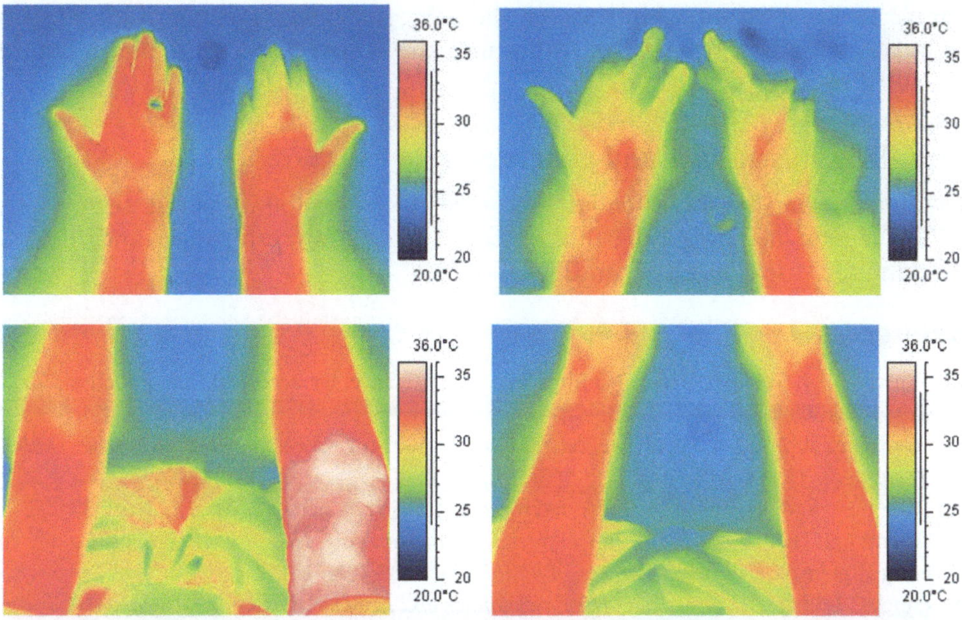

(a) (b)

Figure 21.2. Thermal images of the upper limbs where there are AVF problems. In (*a*) for a patient (female, 43 years) with a brachial AVF there is clear relative warmth on the right upper arm but the fingers on the right hand are clearly colder than the contralateral side hand giving evidence for vascular steal. AVF blood flow was 1780 ml min^{-1}. In (*b*) for a patient (male, 79 years) with a forearm AVF there is no clear area of warmth associated with a patient's fistula giving evidence that this was occluded. Colour duplex ultrasound imaging confirmed the occlusion in this case since blood flow was only 30 ml min^{-1}. Note in (*b*) that the fingers of both hands are generally cool. Reproduced with permission from [6]. Copyright 2006 IOP Publishing.

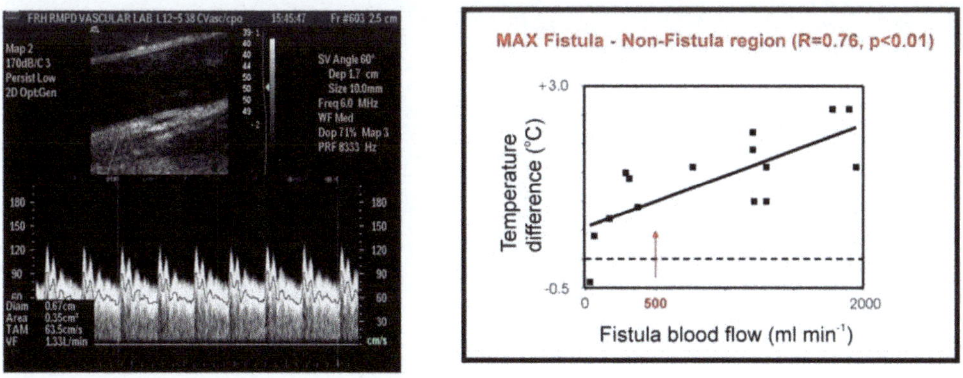

(a) (b)

Figure 21.3. Comparator ultrasound measurements. (*a*) Duplex ultrasound imaging of the fistula. In (*b*) the scatter plot shows a clear and significant relationship between bilateral skin temperature differences on the arm (using the maximum of a chosen region on the AVF side and the non-fistula side) and fistula blood flow measured as by duplex ultrasound. Reproduced with permission from [6]. Copyright IOP Publishing.

significant linear relationship between the degree of bilateral similarity in the arm region temperature around the fistula and the amount of fistula blood flow as measured by duplex ultrasound.

21.4 Brief discussion and conclusion

Thermal imaging has the potential to provide quick and non-invasive assessments of AVF function in terms of fistula patency, blood flow estimation and also for checking for vascular steal from the hand.

References

[1] Murphy G J, White S A and Nicholson M L 2000 Vascular access for haemodialysis *Br. J. Surg.* **87** 1300–01

[2] Rodriguez J A *et al* 2000 The function of permanent vascular access *Nephrol. Dialysis Transplant.* **15** 402–8

[3] Ring E F J and Ammer K 2012 Infrared thermal imaging in medicine *Physiol. Meas.* **33** R33–46

[4] Allen J and Howell K J 2014 Clinical microvascular imaging: techniques and opportunities for clinical physiological measurements *Physiol. Meas.* **35** R91–141

[5] Oates C P 2001 *Cardiovascular Haemodynamics and Doppler Waveforms Explained* (London: Greenwich Medical Media)

[6] Allen J, Oates C P, Chishti A D, Ahmed I A M, Talbot D and Murray A 2006 Thermography and colour duplex ultrasound assessments of arterio-venous fistula function in renal patients *Physiol. Meas.* **27** 51–60

IOP Publishing

Infrared Imaging
A casebook in clinical medicine
Anna Jung, Janusz Żuber, Bolesław Kalicki, Piotr Murawski, Rafał Kuligowski, Ryszard Grenda and Katarzyna Jobs

Chapter 22

Thermographic monitoring of blood flow in arterio-venous fistulas

Maintaining the permeability of arterio-venous fistulas (AVFs) is an important task in haemodialysis patients. In addition to the clinical observation of the fistula, Doppler ultrasonography is used in critical situations. Thermographic examination provides a technique to determine, with high accuracy, the limitations or lack of permeability when it occurs. It is also helpful in monitoring the quality of flow. See figures 22.1–22.3 for examples.

doi:10.1088/978-0-7503-1143-4ch22

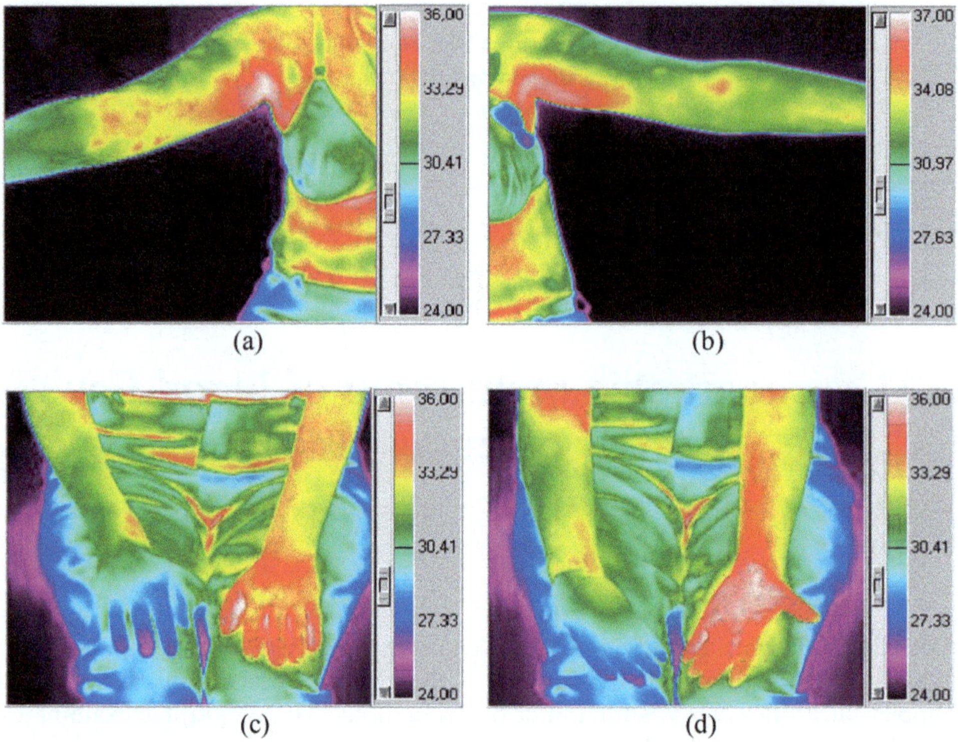

Figure 22.1. Thermograms of the upper limbs of a patient (DW) with haemodialysis fistulas. On the right side the hypothermal area corresponding to circulatory disturbances is clearly visible. (*a*) Upper right arm with a haemodialysis fistula with circulatory disturbances, (*b*) upper left arm with a haemodialysis fistula without circulatory disturbances, (*c*) dorsal palm, hypothermal area on the right palm and (*d*) upper palm, hypothermal area on the right palm.

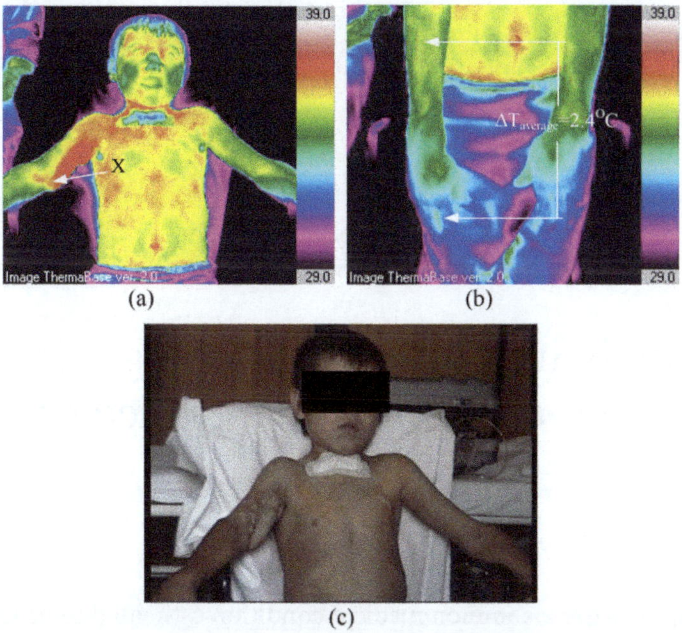

Figure 22.2. Thermograms and a visual image of an AVF in the upper right arm. (*a*) Thermogram with the place of the fistula fold, (*b*) a thermogram demonstrating the difference of temperature between the point of the forearm and the point of the right hand, $\Delta T = 2.4$ °C, and (*c*) a visual image.

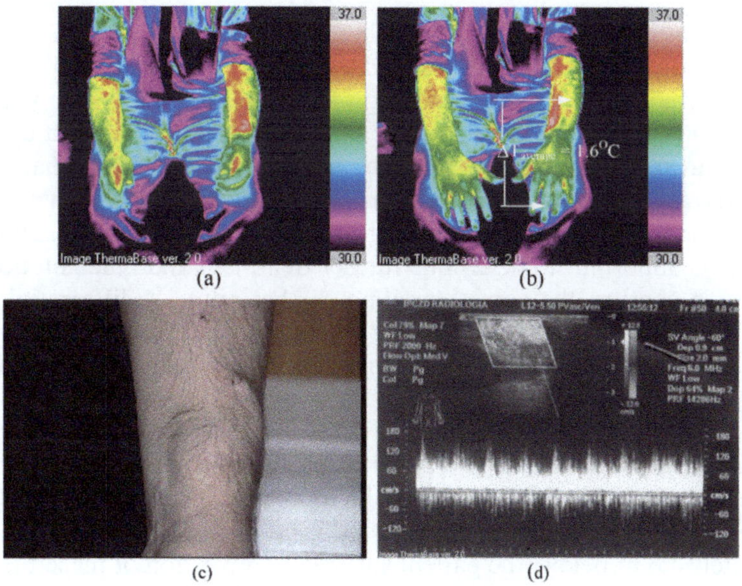

Figure 22.3. Thermograms, a visual image and an image from a Doppler ultrasonography examination of AVFs in the upper left arm in patient MP. (*a*) A thermogram with the AVF on the left upper arm, (*b*) a thermogram showing the difference of temperature between the point of the forearm and the point of the right hand, $\Delta T = 1.6$ °C, (*c*) a visual image of the AVF and (*d*) an image from the AVF ultrasonography examination.

João Oliveira, Ricardo Vardasca, Madalena Pimenta, Joaquim Gabriel and João Torres

Chapter 23

A case study in the diagnosis of a grade III ankle sprain using a combination of medical images

Ankle joint sprains are a common medical condition estimated to be responsible for 15–25% of all musculoskeletal injuries worldwide. The pathophysiology of the lesion can pose considerable time lost to injury, as well as long-term disability in up to 60% of patients. Furthermore, between 10–20% of cases may be complicated by chronic instability of the ankle joint and disability in walking, contributing to morbidity and poor life quality.

Ankle sprains can be classified as grade I, II or III, ranging from mild to severe (I to III) based on the extent of damage and the number of ligaments affected. A grade I sprain is characterized by the stretching of the anterior talofibular and calcaneofibular ligaments. In a grade II sprain, the anterior talofibular ligament tears partially and the calcaneofibular ligament stretches. A grade III sprain is characterized by rupture of the anterior talofibular and calcaneofibular ligaments, with partial tearing of the posterior talofibular and tibiofibular ligaments. An adequate diagnosis in these three grades is important to determine further treatment and rehabilitation.

In order to confirm the correct grading of the injury, a differential diagnostic investigation was performed by verifying the damage of the ankle structures using x-ray and ultrasound images, and thermal images to assess the blood flow and inflammation state.

A 27-year-old male patient, with a BMI of 23.8, conscious, oriented and alert, and in good physical condition presented to the emergency service of Hospital São João. Based on the patient information, the injury had occurred 2 h prior to arrival at the emergency area. While carrying a load from a platform to another positioned approximately 1.5 m below, the patient suffered an inversion of the left foot and fell to the ground. The accompanying symptoms immediately after were acute pain in and proximal to the injury site and progressive swelling and stiffness of the joint.

No ice was placed in the injured area nor were non-steroidal anti-inflammatory drugs administered post-injury. In the objective examination, the ankle joint of the

doi:10.1088/978-0-7503-1143-4ch23

left foot exhibited oedema, stiffness and resistance to mobilization and a slight increase in surface temperature (upon touch when compared to the surrounding skin). The patient presented a blood pressure of SBP/DBP: 123/64 mmHg.

Regarding the patient's past medical history, the patient reported that he had suffered several ankle sprains previously, either in the same or opposite foot, but of which he was unable to define the precise mechanism or approximate point in time. The patient denied alcohol or smoking habits, or elevated blood pressure and other relevant chronic diseases.

The patient exhibited dominance of the right foot. Regarding physical exercise, he stated that he practices with an all-terrain bike three times a week with a 3–4 h practice duration.

After admission the patient was consulted by an orthopaedist and sent for x-ray examination, followed by a thermal physiology assessment using a thermal camera, FLIR E60sc (with a resolution of 320 × 240, a precision of 50 mK and an accuracy of ±2% of the overall reading), the final medical imaging exam used ultrasound performed by a trained physician.

The thermal images were taken in an acclimatized room at 22 °C and a relative humidity of <50% and the patient was placed 1 m from the camera.

No ointments or creams had been applied to the injury area prior to the collection of the data. The patient stated that fasting had begun 3 h 30 min before admission to the emergency area and within this period no coffee, tea, smoking or pharmaceuticals were taken. The patient reported that he had taken an oral dose of Montelukast (a leukotriene receptor antagonist) the night before prior to sleeping. The subject rested for a period of 15 min before the thermal images were taken.

Both ankles were included in the frontal view (figure 23.1) and the thermographic values of the two ankles were compared and assessed through thermal symmetry and

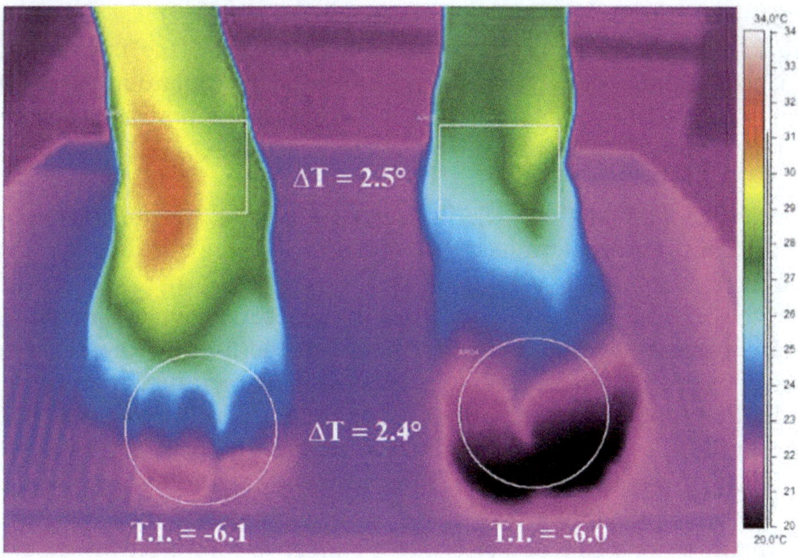

Figure 23.1. The thermal image of the ankles in frontal view, with the thermal symmetry and thermal indexes values.

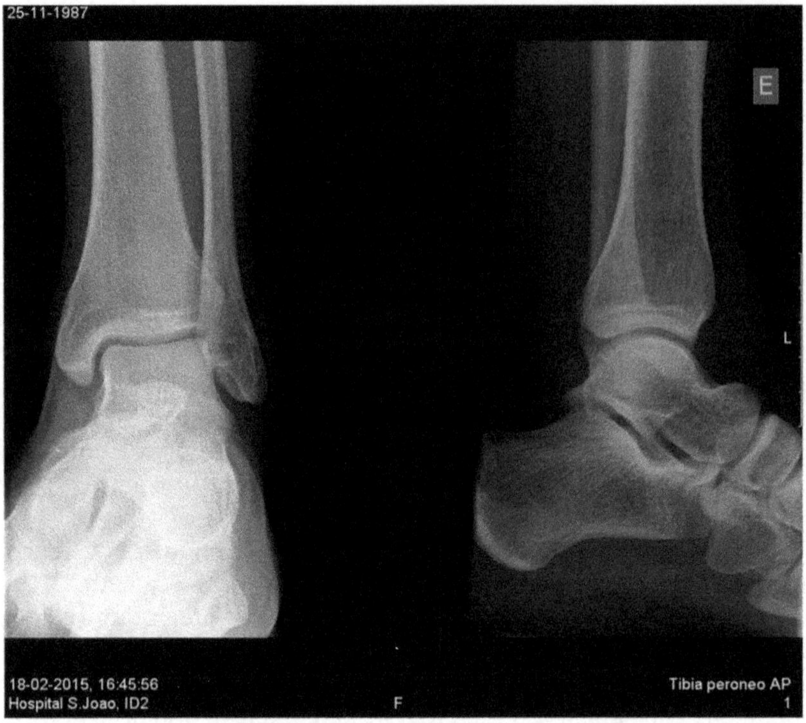

Figure 23.2. Radiographic incidences of the left ankle: frontal and lateral.

a thermal gradient. The thermal symmetry value observed in the affected region of interest was 2.5 °C and the thermal index calculated between the distal region of the foot (phalanges) and the affected area (extensor retinaculum) was –6.0.

Figure 23.2 presents the radiographic images taken in the frontal and lateral incidence, confirming the ligament rupture. The examination was conducted according to the Ottawa guidelines in order to rule out fracture. The results presented in figure 23.2 do not show any evidence of complete or partial bone fracture.

Finally, ultrasound analysis was in agreement with the previous clinical and imaging findings and determined the extent of ligament damage and joint compromise.

Injuries to the ankle joints, such as ankle sprains, can provoke thermal variations leading to either hypothermia or hyperthermia of the foot and nearby anatomical areas. The above described case shows a decrease in temperature between the injured and non-injured foot of more than 2 °C. The thermal profile observed in this case might be similar to other cases of ankle joint sprains and be useful for comparison, and potentially associated, with the clinical diagnosis grading and other imaging analysis. It should be highlighted that if a correlation is shown and the grading of ankle sprain lesions can be performed or aided by infrared thermography, its clinical application has several advantages. This technique is non-invasive and does not involve contact with the lesion site and therefore does not impose further pain on the patient. Thermography can deliver information in real time and does not require a highly specialized technician to perform the initial evaluation. In addition infrared thermographic equipment is more affordable to most clinical units and individual physicians involved in sports medicine. It is portable and may be a valuable tool in the diagnosis of acute ankle joint lesions in different scenarios.

IOP Publishing

Infrared Imaging
A casebook in clinical medicine
Ricardo Vardasca, Ana Domingues and Joaquim Gabriel

Chapter 24

Thermal imaging in the monitoring of grade III ankle sprain rehabilitation—a case study

Ankle sprain is the most frequent injury affecting the lower limbs and it is often regarded as trivial, not having a simple, objective and accurate diagnosis and treatment evaluation. This condition occurs when the ankle rolls outward and the foot turns inward, resulting in stretching and tearing of the ligaments on the outside of the ankle, or when the ankle rolls inward and the foot turns outward, damaging the ligaments on the inside of the ankle. Ankle sprains can be classified into three grades, which can range from stretching (grade I) to partial rupture (grade II) or to complete rupture of the ligament (grade III).

It is known that ankle sprains, accompanied by tenderness, swelling and stiffness, are associated with pain and inflammation. Temperature changes associated with the inflammatory process can be monitored by medical thermal imaging.

A male subject, a rugby player of 18 years of age and a BMI of 24.5, suffered a grade III ankle sprain in the left ankle, with a complete rupture of the anterior talofibular and calcaneofibular ligaments, which was confirmed by other imaging examinations (x-ray and ultrasound) at the Hospital São João. The subject was totally immobilized for 20 days before receiving physiotherapy.

A FLIR A325sc thermal camera (with a resolution of 320×240, a precision of 70 mK and an accuracy of $\pm 2\%$ of the overall reading) was used to collect the thermal images in an acclimatized room at 19 °C and a relative humidity of $<60\%$. The subject was placed 70 cm away from the camera, which was mounted on a tripod.

Figure 24.1 shows the regions of interest (ROIs) used to monitor the affected areas in the three different views.

Thermograms of both ankles were captured after an acclimatization period of 15 min and before the first physiotherapy session (figure 24.2—day 1). They showed evidence of increased temperature in the injured ankle. The difference in the temperatures recorded in both ankles was obvious in both the frontal and lateral views.

doi:10.1088/978-0-7503-1143-4ch24

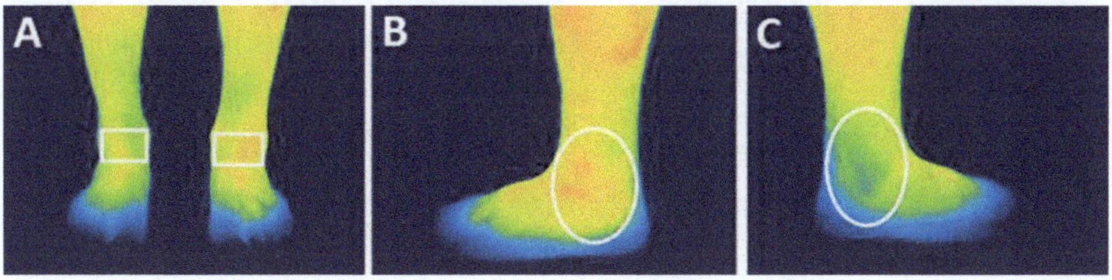

Figure 24.1. Views: (*A*) frontal, (*B*) lateral left and (*C*) lateral right.

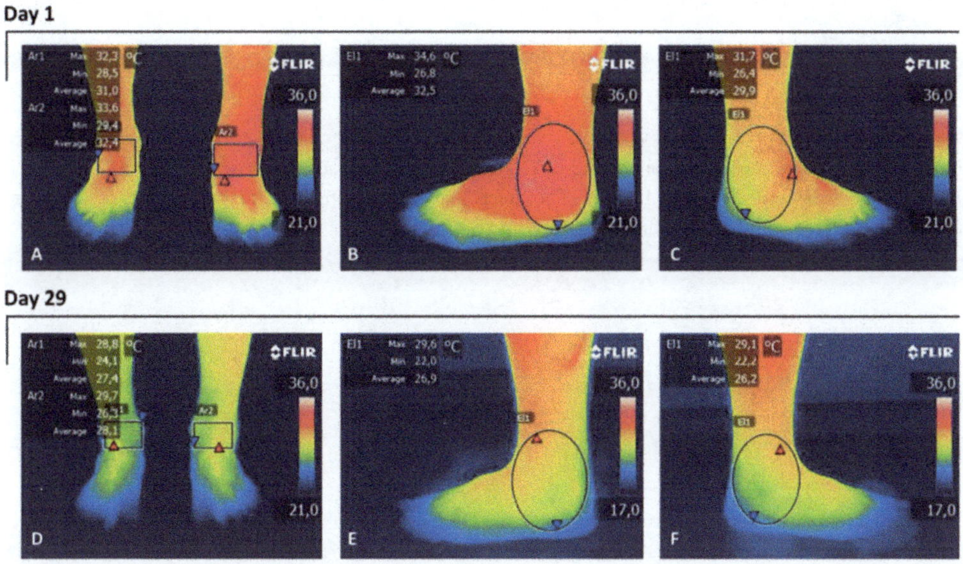

Figure 24.2. Thermal images on different day of examination (1st and 29th day of treatment). (*A*) Frontal view (day 1), (*B*) left lateral view (day 1), (*C*) right lateral view (day 1), (*D*) frontal view (day 29), (*E*) left lateral view (day 29) and (*F*) right lateral view (day 29).

Treatment consisted of 20 min immersion in an ice bucket, which was followed by Thera-Band exercises (dorsiflexion, plantarflexion, inversion and eversion) for 5 min per session. The subject abstained from sport (did not return to practice) during the follow-up period.

There was a clear reduction in temperature difference, due to the decrease in the mean temperature of the ROIs of the injured ankle, indicating a decrease in inflammation. The progress in recovery is documented by the thermograms (figure 24.2—day 29).

The temperature course in the frontal and lateral views were different (figure 24.3). In the frontal thermograms, the temperature difference was resolved at day 16, became borderline on day 25 and was slightly abnormal at the last examination. In the lateral view the temperature difference was only almost resolved on day 29.

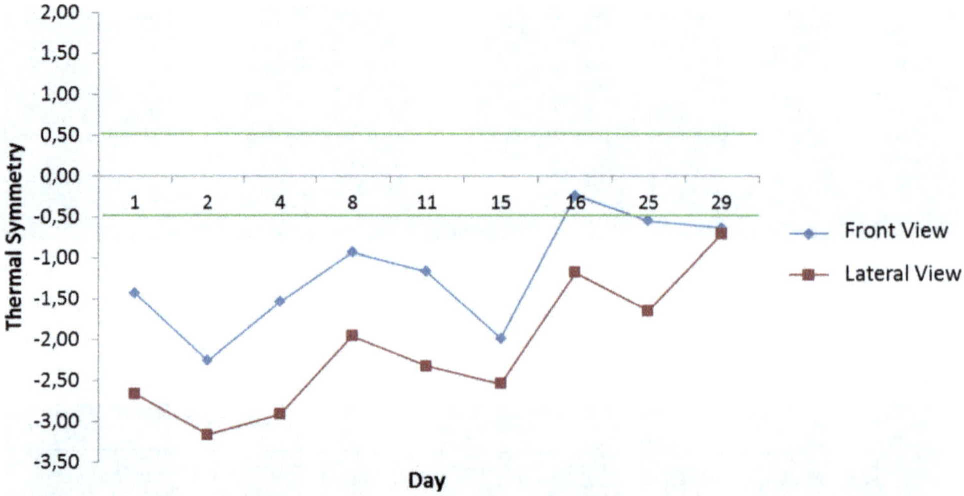

Figure 24.3. Graphic representation of the ankle temperature differences during the rehabilitation period (blue: frontal view and red: lateral view). The green line indicates the arbitrary threshold of the normal temperature difference of corresponding anatomical sites.

IOP Publishing

Infrared Imaging
A casebook in clinical medicine
B. Kalicki, A. Lipińska-Opałka, A. Krawczyk, A. Jung, J. Żuber, J. Mróz

Chapter 25

Application of thermal imaging in the diagnosis and treatment monitoring of complex regional pain syndrome type I

Complex regional pain syndrome (CRPS) is a chronic condition caused by inflammatory and sympathetic nervous dysfunction. It is characterized by severe pain of the distal part of limbs, oedema, vasomotor dysfunction and impaired efficiency. These symptoms occur after different types of trauma. Limb pain and swelling, in typical cases, are accompanied by vasomotor disturbances, restricted mobility, increased sensitivity to pressure and temperature changes. The effectiveness of treatment depends on the period in which the diagnosis is made. The sooner patients are treated, the better are the outcomes. There are no specific diagnostic tests that can establish reliable diagnosis in patients suspected of having CRPS. Imaging studies are useful in the diagnosis.

A 42-year-old man, several weeks after arthroscopy of the left knee, came to an orthopaedic surgeon with pain and swelling of the ankle and left foot. After radiography of the left foot, the patient received treatment for gouty arthritis. Despite the treatment the pain was not reduced. USG of the left foot showed swelling of the synovial membrane with massive hyperaemia and Doppler USG showed the correct picture of arterial and venous vessels. The conclusion of MRI was a non-specific image, suggesting CRPS. The patient was referred to the Rehabilitation Centre of the Military Institute of Medicine, where thermographic investigation showed a significant temperature difference between the sick and healthy foot (5.7 °C). Long-term physical therapy was undertaken achieving clinical improvement, decrease of the oedema and reduction in pain. The whole treatment process was monitored using thermography (see figures 25.1 and 25.2).

doi:10.1088/978-0-7503-1143-4ch25

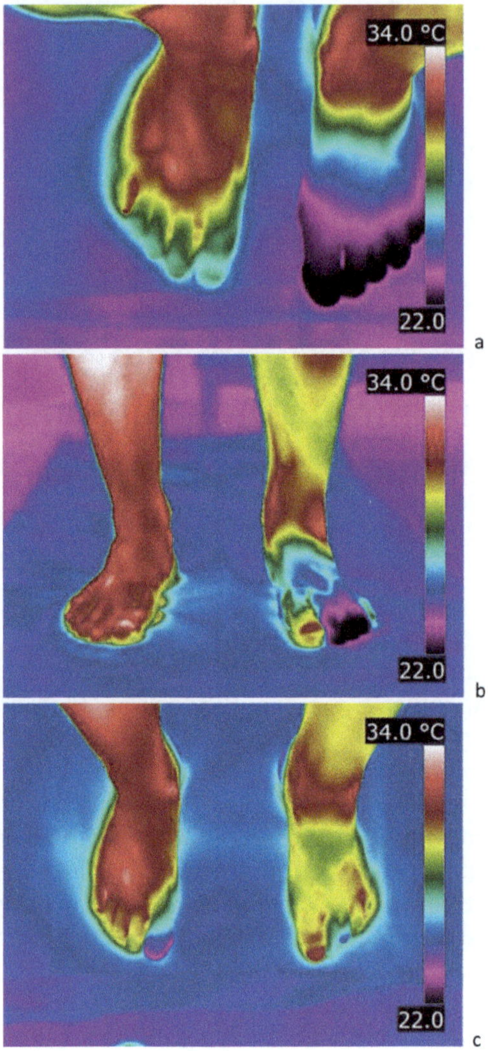

Figure 25.1. Thermography of the feet. (*a*) Before treatment: the temperature difference between the sick and healthy foot was 5.7 °C. (*b*) After 20 d of therapy: the temperature difference between the sick and healthy foot was 2.0 °C. (*c*) After 6 weeks of therapy: the temperature difference between the sick and healthy foot was 1.2 °C.

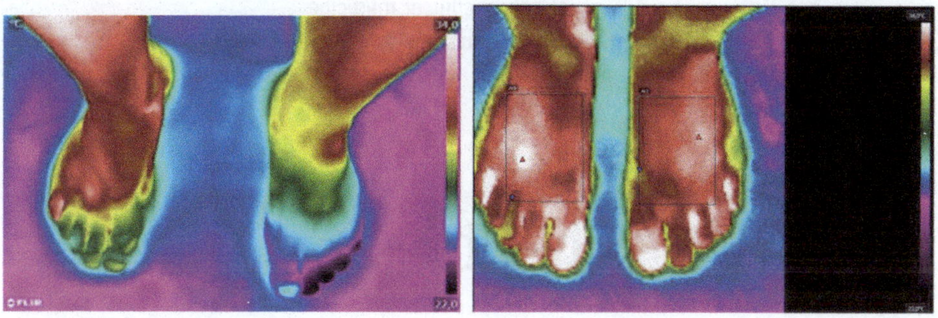

a. b.

Figure 25.2. Thermography of the feet. (*a*) After 2 months without any physical therapy: the temperature difference between the sick and healthy foot was 3.2 °C. (*b*) After 20 d of magnetotherapy: the temperature difference between the sick and healthy foot was 0.2 °C.

Chapter 26

The thermal imaging potential for assessing diabetic Charcot foot syndrome

26.1 Description

Charcot neuropathic osteoarthropathy [1] has been documented to occur as a consequence of various peripheral neuropathies; however, diabetic neuropathy has become the most common aetiology. The interaction of several component factors results in an acute localized inflammatory condition that may lead to varying degrees and patterns of bone destruction, subluxation, dislocation and deformity.

Current assessments in the clinic can include spot infrared thermometry skin temperature measurements to detect local elevations in tissue temperature. This can be time consuming to carry out. This case study reports the application of thermal imaging [2] to a patient presenting clinically with a very high risk of Charcot's. Thermography has the potential to enhance clinical assessment in this patient group as it could help identify and communicate, with confidence, regions of inflammation associated with the condition [3].

26.2 Clinical presentation

A 36-year-old female diabetic patient with a known Charcot joint at the left ankle is presented in this case study.

26.3 Investigations and procedures, diagnostic findings

Lower limb thermography was performed at Freeman Hospital's Microvascular Diagnostics measurement facility. The patient followed the pre-imaging protocol instructions which included avoiding any smoking, caffeinated substances and talc/creams on the skin of the feet on the day of their test. They arrived at the hospital and were acclimatized for at least 10 min in the temperature controlled room for imaging at the normothermic room setting (23 °C). A thermal imaging camera (FLIR Systems SC300) was used with measurements made with the subject supine.

doi:10.1088/978-0-7503-1143-4ch26

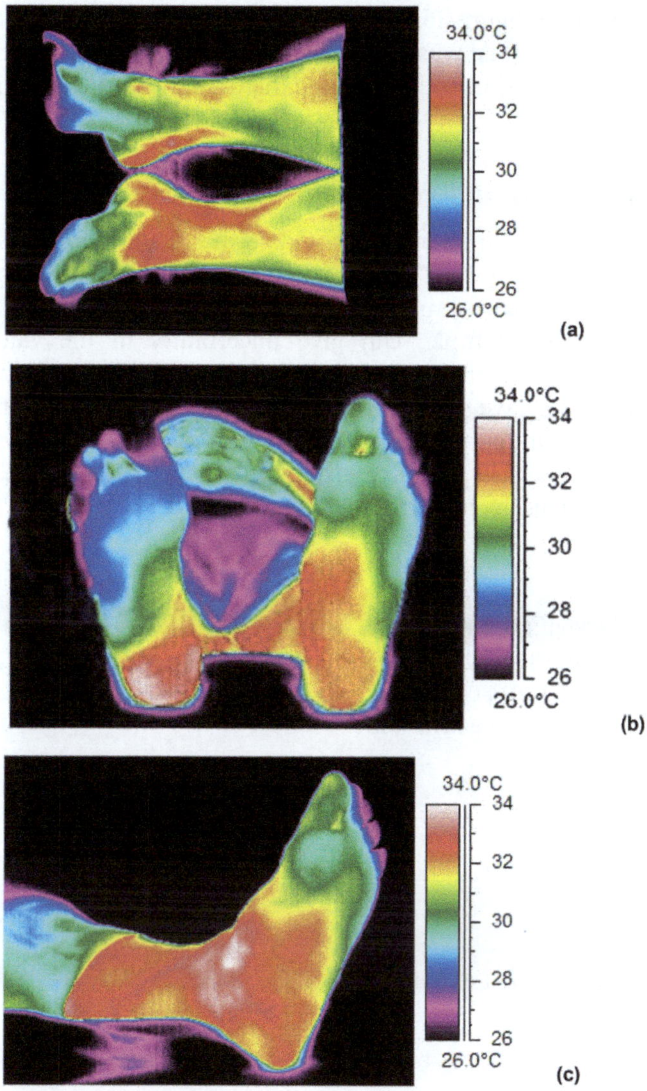

Figure 26.1. Thermal image of the left foot of a patient presenting clinically with known Charcot's at the left ankle joint. The elevated temperatures and their localization across the foot are clear from these three views (*a*)–(*c*). There are also warm areas at the right heel area and extending into the medial ankle aspect but this was attributed on clinical assessment to very dry skin and associated inflammation. Care is therefore needed when contrasting bilateral temperature differences and with image interpretation when multiple pathologies might be present.

Thermograms were visualized using dedicated image processing software (FLIR ThermaCam Researcher, skin emissivity = 0.98) with a 'rainbow scale' across a temperature range of 8 °C.

Bilateral temperature differences were seen between the feet with left–right thermal asymmetries greater than +1 °C at the ankle joint, the average in areas for three views (anterior, medial and plantar). The maximum focal bilateral difference was greater than +2 °C (figures 26.1(*a*)–(*c*)). The deformity with tissue swelling at the medial left ankle aspect is evident in figure 26.1(*b*). In addition, the heel of the right foot and into the medial aspect of the ankle was clearly warmer than the contralateral side but this was attributed to very dry skin and associated inflammation on clinical presentation at the measurement session.

26.4 Brief discussion and conclusion

Thermal imaging has the capability to provide a quick and non-invasive assessment of the degree of inflammation in Charcot joints in patients with diabetes. The case study also highlights that care in image interpretation is very important as co-existent skin inflammation, for example, can give uncertainty in the value of bilateral temperature differences. Furthermore, the study also highlights that thermal imaging of the whole foot may have greater clinical utility compared to using just a small number of localized spot temperatures made by non-imaging spot temperature probe devices; further assessment in a defined group of diabetic patients with Charcot joints would be needed to help demonstrate this.

References

[1] Rogers L C *et al* 2011 The Charcot foot in diabetes *Diabetes Care* **34** 2123–9

[2] Ring E F J and Ammer K 2012 Infrared thermal imaging in medicine *Physiol. Meas.* **33** R33–46

[3] Allen J and Howell K J 2014 Clinical microvascular imaging: techniques and opportunities for clinical physiological measurements *Physiol. Meas.* **35** R91–141

IOP Publishing

Infrared Imaging
A casebook in clinical medicine
Ricardo Vardasca, Ana Marques, Rui Carvalho and Joaquim Gabriel

Chapter 27

Thermal imaging of the foot in different forms of diabetic disease

Diabetes affects around 8.3% of the world population and one in seven patients are at a high risk of developing diabetic foot problems. This condition involves several anatomic-pathological and peripheral neurological disorders which affect peripheral microcirculation. This can have serious consequences such as ulcers, ischemia and amputation. A practical and inexpensive monitoring and assessment tool is needed for evaluating treatments progression and to act promptly in the case of regression.

Medical thermography was used to monitor the temperature distribution on the plantar feet view, following a standard capture protocol. This information is directly related with the physiology, allowing for real-time physiological assessment, providing a window on the peripheral microvascular and autonomic nervous systems, which are directly related with the pathology. A total of 50 patients were investigated, 30 neuropathic, 2 ischemic and 18 neuroischaemic. Regions of interest (ROIs) for the plantar view of the feet (figure 27.1) were defined in the most common locations of diabetic foot ulcers.

The thermal images of the plantar feet were taken using the set up described in figure 27.2 in an acclimatized room (mean temperature 22 ± 1 °C and a relative humidity of <50%) after the patient had undergone a 15 min period of thermal equilibration. A FLIR A325sc thermal camera (with a resolution of 320×240, a precision of 70 mK and an accuracy of ±2% of the overall reading) mounted on a tripod was used. The patients were placed 70 cm from the camera.

The diabetic foot can be of three types: neuropathic, ischaemic or neuroischaemic, an example thermal image of each is shown in figure 27.3.

Examining the results obtained for the three types of diabetic foot per each defined ROI, it can be observed in this sample, that the ischemic cases have higher thermal symmetry at the A2, A3, A4, A6 and A8, the neuropathic cases at the Al and A7 and the neuroischaemic at the A9 and A10 ROIs (figure 27.4).

doi:10.1088/978-0-7503-1143-4ch27

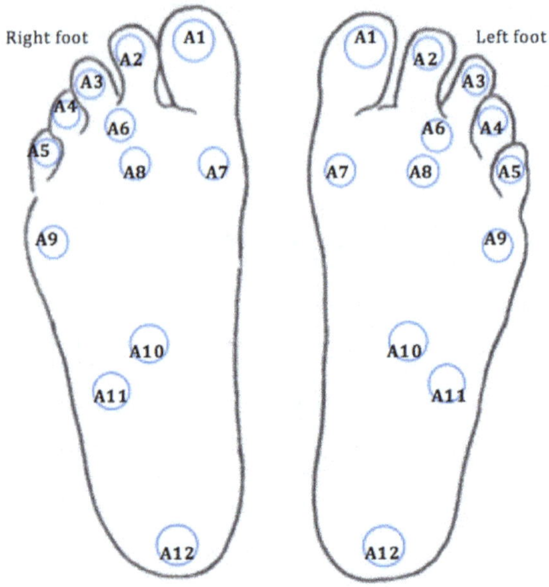

Figure 27.1. Definition of ROIs for assessing the VS (left) and ANS (right) of the feet.

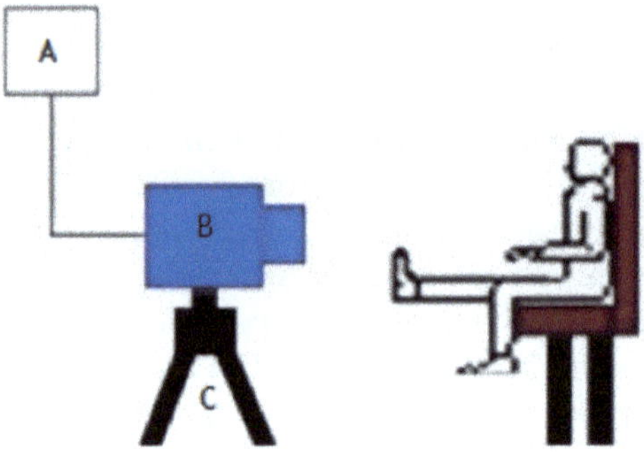

Figure 27.2. Thermal image capture set up (*A*: laptop; *B*: thermal camera; and *C*: tripod).

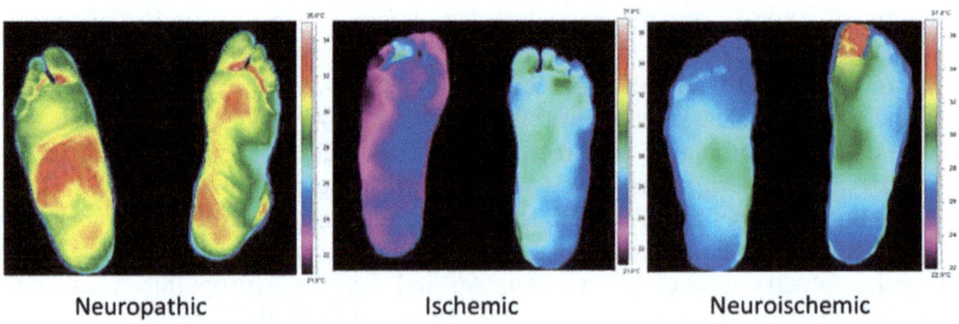

Figure 27.3. Example thermal images of the three types of diabetic foot.

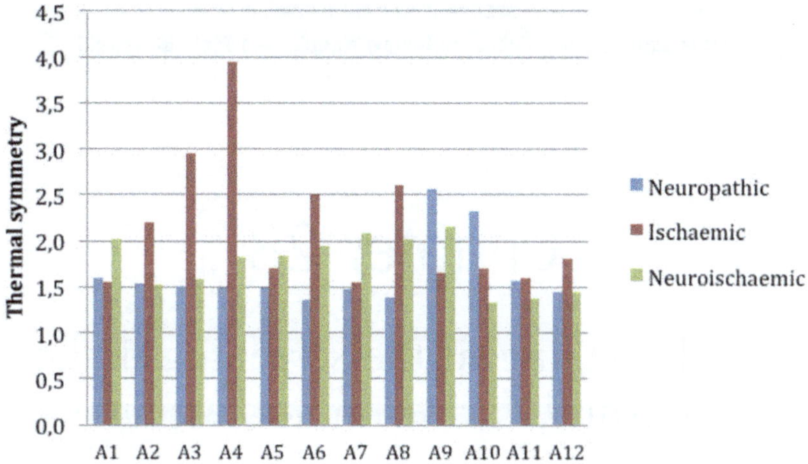

Figure 27.4. Comparison of the three types of diabetic foot per ROI defined for the ANS (left) and the VS (right).

The results of this study proved useful in studying diabetic foot disease more extensively and improving our knowledge of its pathophysiology. The use of thermography confirmed the influence that the type of diabetes, blood glucose level, BMI and age have on the clinical condition.

The results obtained are of potential value as a reference. This proposed methodology can be improved for use in daily practice. It could therefore be of value in the diagnosis and treatment assessment for the provision of improved clinical management and reduction in associated healthcare costs.

IOP Publishing

Infrared Imaging
A casebook in clinical medicine
Anna Jung, Janusz Żuber, Bolesław Kalicki and Piotr Murawski

Chapter 28

Thermal imaging in the screening diagnosis of crural varices in adolescents

Pathology of the venous system poses a significant danger of thrombus formation and its complications. Early detection and rapid diagnosis are two important factors in the problem of crural varices in adolescents. Abnormalities of the venous system can occur in the early period of life. In addition to the usual clinical identification, there are other diagnostic imaging methods which should be applied. Doppler ultrasonography is the preferred choice, since other methods of venous-flow imaging are invasive.

The aim of this study was to assess the role of thermal imaging as an adjunct in the screening examination of varicose veins of the lower limbs.

Thermal imaging examination was performed in 44 young, healthy people (25–38 years old, 38 females and 6 males) using an Inframetrics ThermaCAM SC1000 camera and a digital photographic camera (see figures 28.1–28.9).

The following quantitative parameters of the thermograms were measured:

- maximum temperature,
- median temperature,
- Δ (the temperature difference between images of two different areas of the same limb or both limbs) and
- standard deviation (SD).

The patient results were divided into two groups depending on the presence of changes in the thermogram. 8/44 (13.6%) patients with visible abnormalities in the thermographic image were classified in the I group.

The other patients, 36/44 (86.4%), were classified in the II group on the basis of a symmetric thermographic image of the lower limbs, without significant hypo- or hyperthermal areas.

In the physical and photographic (digital camera) examinations all patients showed no abnormalities in the peripheral venous system of the lower limbs.

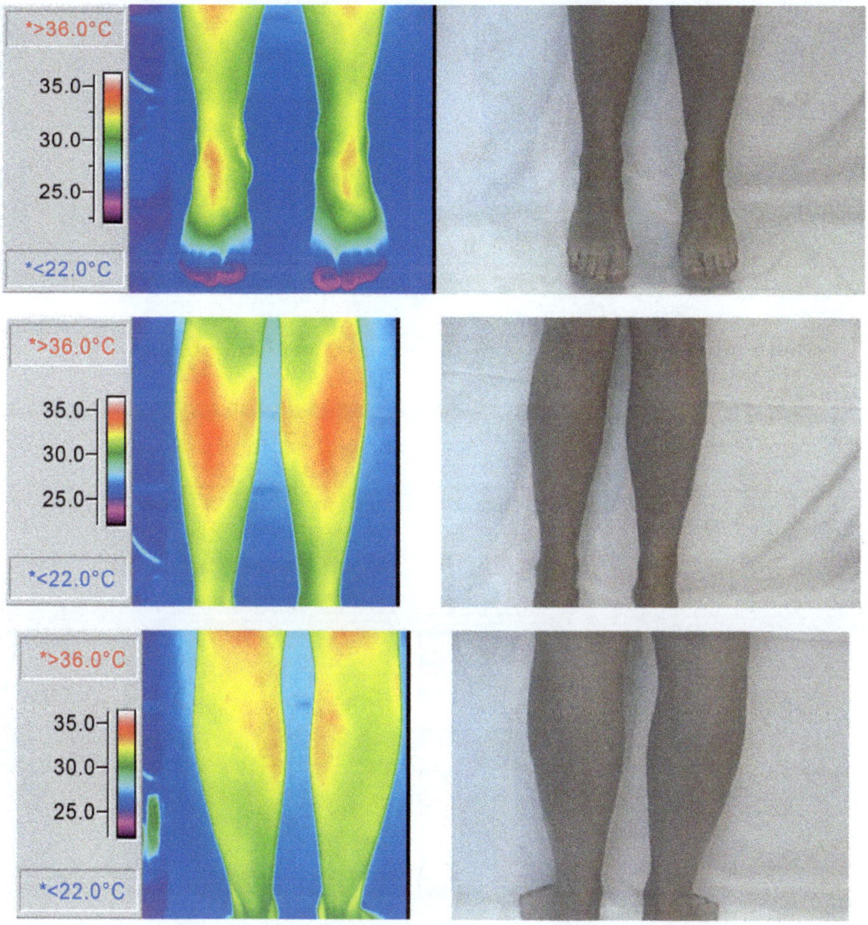

Figure 28.1. Thermographic and visual images of the lower limbs of 28-year-old female patient ES.

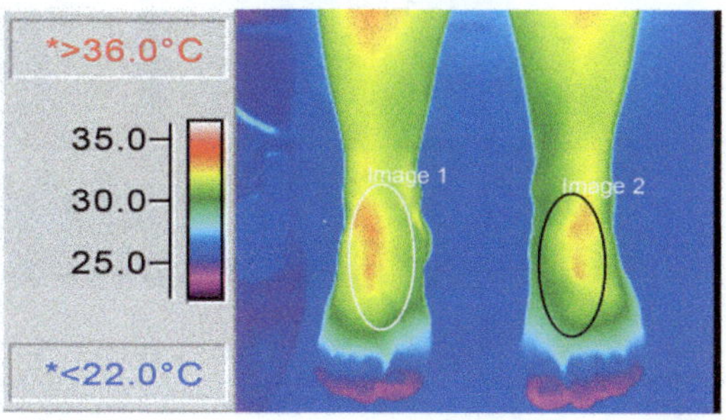

Temperature index	T_{Image1}	T_{Image2}	$\Delta(T_{\text{Image1}} - T_{\text{Image2}})$
Minimum	27.6	27.6	0.0
Maximum	33.4	33.0	0.4
Average	31.2	30.9	0.3
Media	31.5	31.0	0.5
SD	1.2	1.2	

Figure 28.2. Thermogram and thermal parameters of the lower limbs of ES.

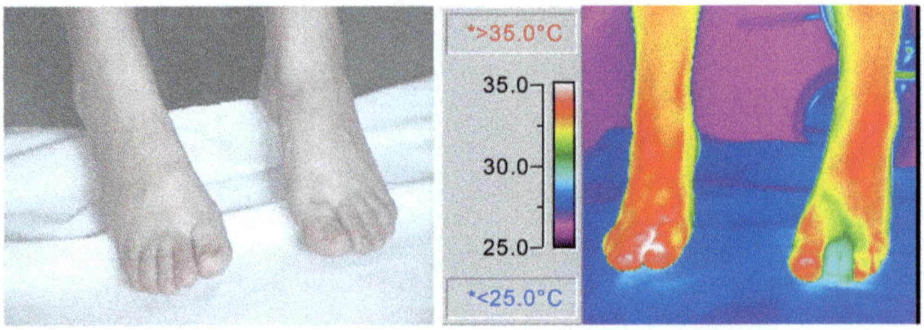

Temperature index	T_{Image1}	T_{Image2}	$\Delta(T_{Image1} - T_{Image2})$
Minimum	28.7	28.5	0.2
Maximum	34.8	33.0	1.8
Average	33.2	29.8	3.4
Median	33.2	29.5	3.7
SD	0.6	0.9	

Figure 28.3. Visual and thermographic images and thermal parameters of the lower limbs of female patient IW.

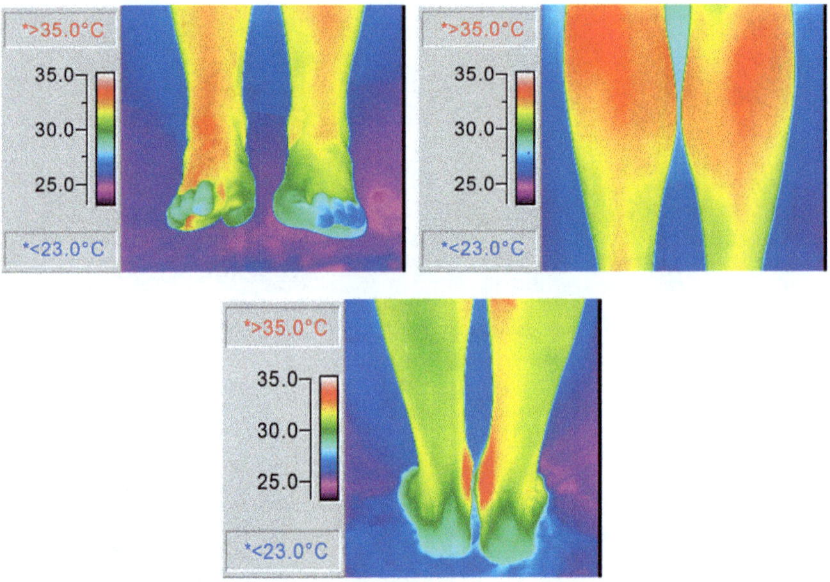

Temperature index	T_{Image1}	T_{Image2}	$\Delta(T_{Image1} - T_{Image2})$
Minimum	26.5	25.8	0.7
Maximum a	31.6	32.7	1.1
Average	29.8	31.1	1.3
Median	30.7	31.8	1.1
SD	1.5	1.5	

Figure 28.4. Thermal images of the lower legs in different aspects.

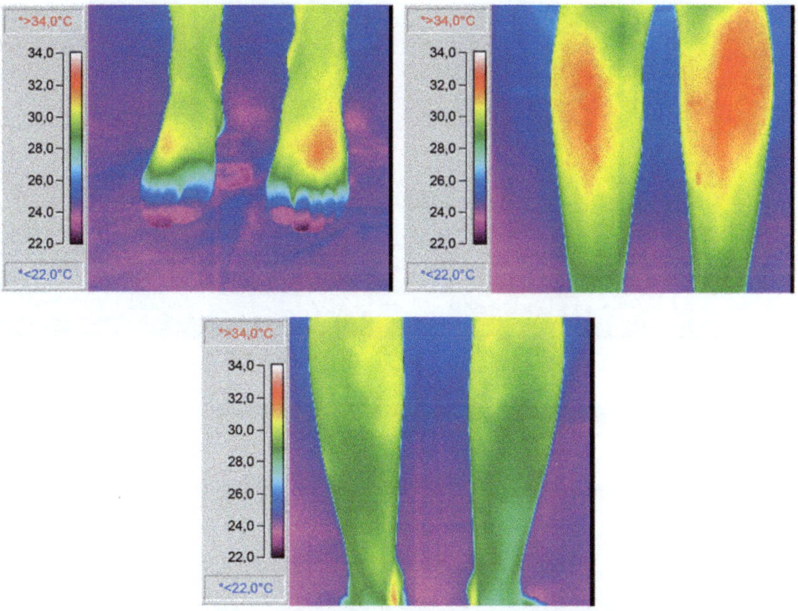

Temperature index	T_{Image1}	T_{Image2}	$\Delta(T_{\mathrm{Image1}} - T_{\mathrm{Image2}})$
Minimum	25.2	24.2	1.0
Maximum	29.3	30.1	0.8
Average	27.3	28.6	1.3
Median	27.4	28.7	1.3
SD	0.9	0.9	

Figure 28.5. Thermal images of the lower legs in different aspects.

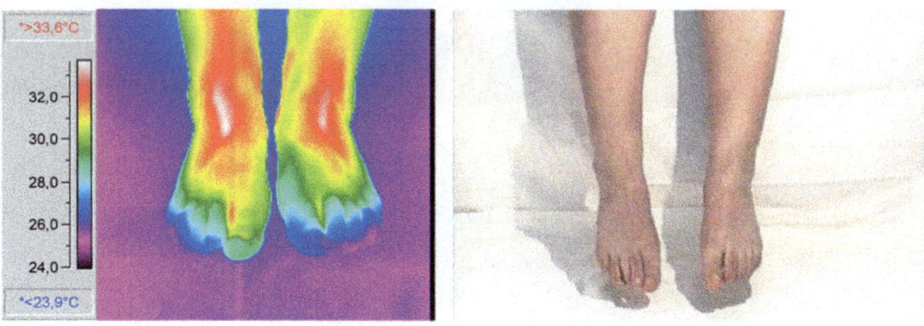

Figure 28.6. Thermographic and visual images of the lower limbs of 25-year-old female patient TB-M.

The thermal imaging investigation allowed us to distinguish two groups of patients. The distinctive criterion was an at least 0.8 °C difference between symmetric limbs. In the I group average temperature changes from 0.97–3.35 °C were obtained giving the mean group value of 1.56 °C, with SD = 0.76 °C. The median (most frequently observed) temperature was from 1.0–3.7 °C, with group mean value = 1.63 °C and SD = 0.87 °C.

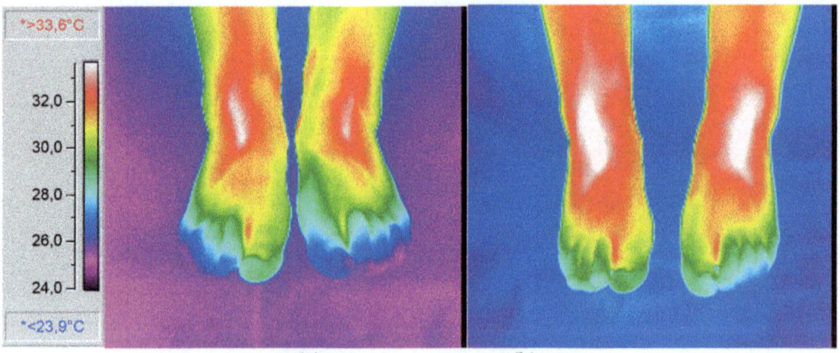

(a) (b)

Thermal indexes (a)

T_{Image1}	T_{Image2}	T_{Image1}	$\Delta(T_{Image1} - T_{Image2})$
Minimum	27.2	1.5	25.7
Maximum	31.8	1.2	30.6
Average	29.9	1.6	28.4
Median	30.2	1.8	28.4
SD	0.9		1.4

Thermal indexes (b)

T_{Image1}	T_{Image2}	T_{Image1}	$\Delta(T_{Image1} - T_{Image2})$
Minimum	25.2	1.0	24.2
Maximum	29.3	0.8	30.1
Average	27.3	1.3	28.6
Median	27.4	1.3	28.7
SD	0.9		0.9

Figure 28.7. Thermograms and thermal indexes (*a*) before treatment and (*b*) 6 weeks after treatment (Xantinol Nicotinate).

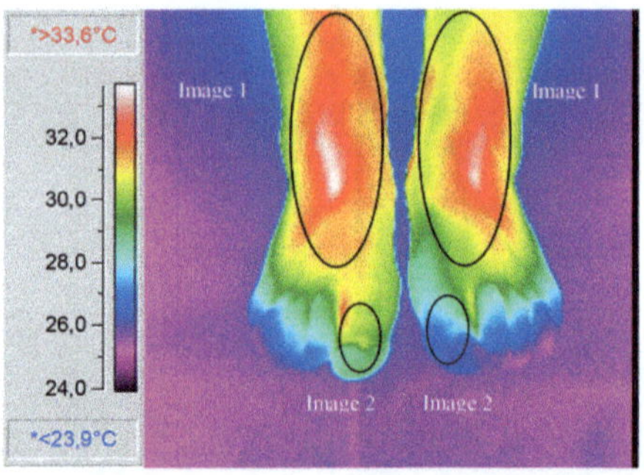

Temperature index	T_{Image1}	T_{Image2}	$\Delta(T_{Image1} - T_{Image2})$
Minimum	28.4	28.5	0.1
Maximum	33.7	30.4	3.3
Average	31.5	29.4	2.1

Temperature index	T_{Image1}	T_{Image2}	$\Delta(T_{Image1} - T_{Image2})$
Minimum	29.6	25.8	3.8
Maximum	33.4	27.1	6.3
Average	31.3	26.2	5.1

Figure 28.8. The thermogram and the value of the thermal indices of the lower limbs of patient TB-M before treatment.

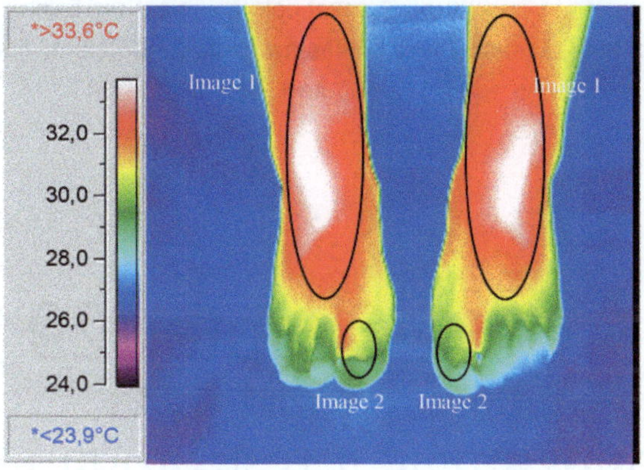

Temperature index	T_{Image1}	T_{Image2}	$\Delta(T_{Image1} - T_{Image2})$
Minimum	29.4	28.8	0.6
Maximum	34.6	31.4	3.2
Average	32.4	29.9	2.5

Temperature index	T_{Image1}	T_{Image2}	$\Delta(T_{Image1} - T_{Image2})$
Minimum	27.6	28.1	0.5
Maximum	34.5	30.5	4.0
Average	31.9	29.2	2.7

Figure 28.9. Thermogram of the lower limbs of patient TB-M and the value of the thermal indices 6 weeks after treatment (Xantinol Nicotinate).

In group II the average temperature changes were from 0.08–0.83 °C, giving a mean group value of 0.44 °C, with SD = 0.23 °C. The median was from 0.0–0.8 °C, with a group mean value of 0.46 °C and SD = 0.27 °C.

These results indicate that thermal imaging is a useful and non-invasive method in the screening examination of the venous system in the lower limbs. The quantitative parameters of the thermograms (maximum temperature, median temperature, SD) provide additional information. It is interesting to note that these results are not dependant on the choice of region of interest in the comparative areas.

IOP Publishing

Infrared Imaging
A casebook in clinical medicine
Anna Jung, Janusz Żuber, Bolesław Kalicki, Wojciech Perdzyński, Marek Klewar and Piotr Murawski

Chapter 29

Thermographic investigation in the diagnosis of femoral vein thrombosis

A 12-year-old boy (GB) was hospitalized at the Clinic of Children's Surgery at the Military School of Medicine following 9 d of fever, pain and oedema of the left thigh. He was visibly limping and when resting, he kept the left hip joint flexed. There were visible dilated veins beneath the skin of the left upper thigh and left buttock. Doppler ultrasound of the femoral vein revealed a thrombus occluding blood flow. The other lower limb veins were patent and arterial flow was normal. Treatment with intravenous antibiotics, fractionized heparin and fibrinolytic medicines (streptase, actylize) was commenced. However the thrombus did not disperse. Long-term anticoagulant therapy was undertaken. The prothrombin level was maintained at 35–45% and the APTT index at 1.70–1.90. Follow-up Doppler ultrasound studies showed partial recanalization and disappearance of the thrombus in the left superficial femoral vein (see figure 29.1). There was a good correlation between the thermographic studies and the Doppler ultrasound images.

doi:10.1088/978-0-7503-1143-4ch29

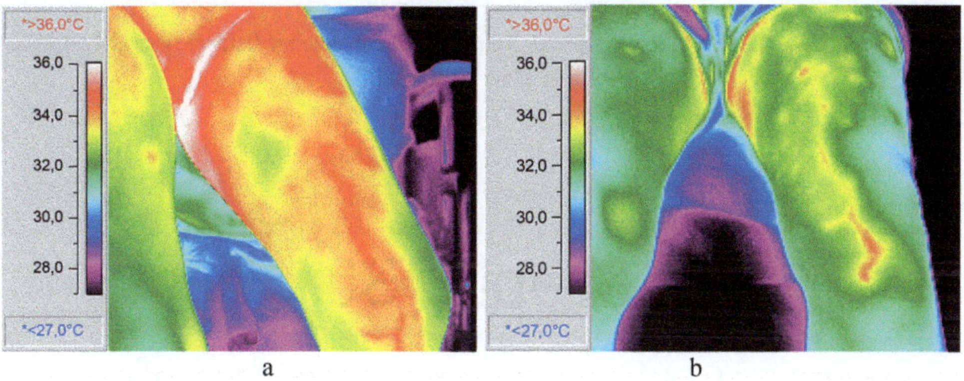

Figure 29.1. Thermographic investigation in the diagnosis of left femoral vein thrombosis. (*a*) Before treatment: hyperthermal area over the left femoral vein, temperature gradient 3.5 °C. (*b*) After treatment: limitation hyperthermal area.

Anna Jung, Janusz Żuber, Bolesław Kalicki, Marek Stańczyk, Michał Osiecki, Paweł Twarkowski and Piotr Murawski

Chapter 30

Infrared thermal imaging of critical leg ischaemia

The case of a 60-year-old female patient (GA) with a 10 year history of arteriosclerosis obliterans with an ischaemic right lower limb, lumbar symphatectomy and successful functioning of a right femoropopliteal prosthesis is presented.

The patient was admitted to the surgical department with symptoms and signs such as pain at rest, muscle stiffness and a distance of intermittent claudication of 50 m. On physical examination trophic changes of the skin of the right lower limb were observed. Doppler ultrasound and angiography confirmed occlusion of the right femoropopliteal prosthesis. The indication for surgical intervention was limb salvage. During the operation an occluded femoropopliteal prosthesis was found. The surgical procedure included restoring the prosthesis patency by embolectomy and profundoplasty with a venous patch above the proximal part of the deep femoral artery. Because there was no evident clinical improvement of the lower limb perfusion, the surgical procedure was followed by 7 d of aloprostadil (Prostavasin, PGE_1) administration. Due to aggravation of the right lower limb ischaemia our patient required below knee amputation. The infrared thermography findings had a strong correlation with the clinical picture (figures 30.1–30.4).

A second case is presented, a patient (BS) with critical leg ischemia. He was treated with good results using aloprostadil (figure 30.5).

doi:10.1088/978-0-7503-1143-4ch30

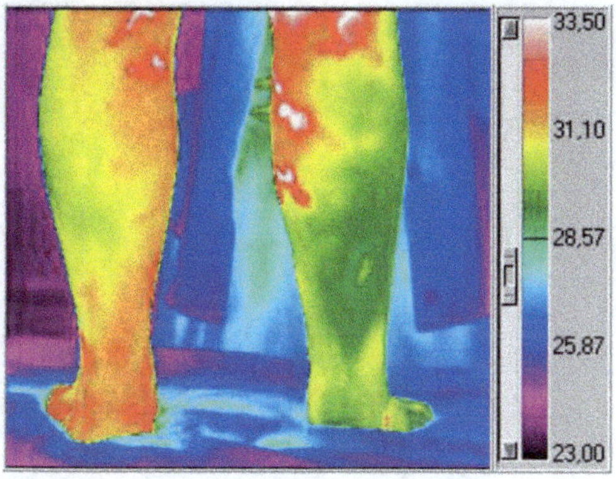

Figure 30.1. Thermogram of the lower limbs before surgery (embolectomy and profundoplasty), patient GA.

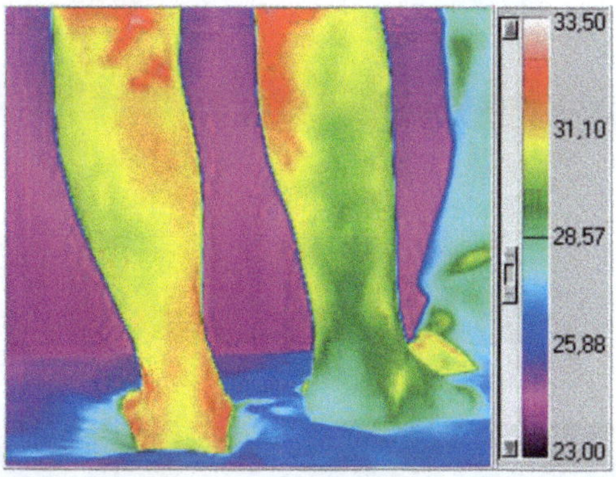

Figure 30.2. Thermogram of the lower limbs after surgery (embolectomy and profundoplasty), patient GA.

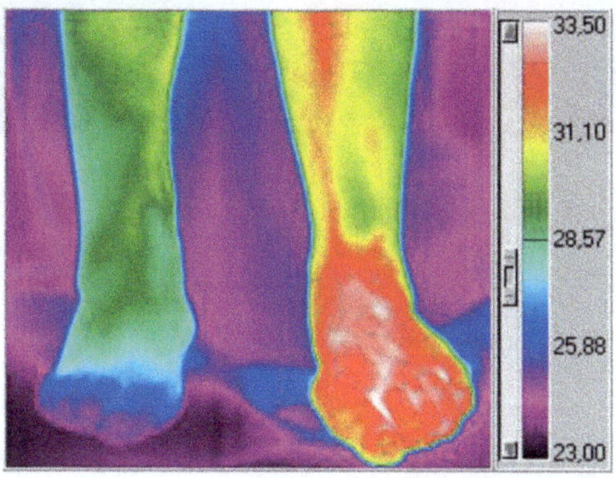

Figure 30.3. Thermogram of the lower limbs after aloprostadil (Prostavasin) administration, patient GA.

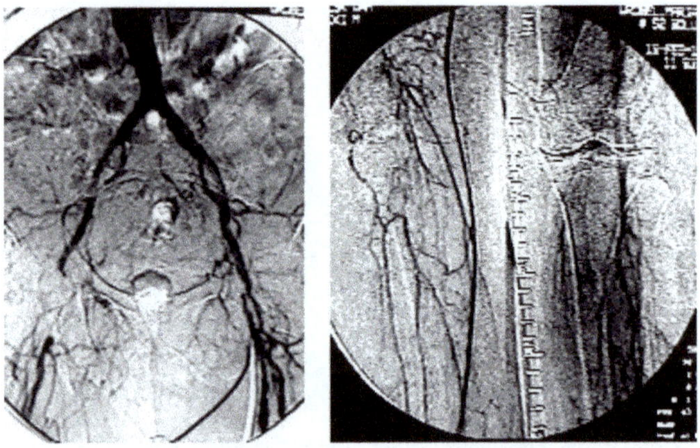

Figure 30.4. Angiography examination, patient GA.

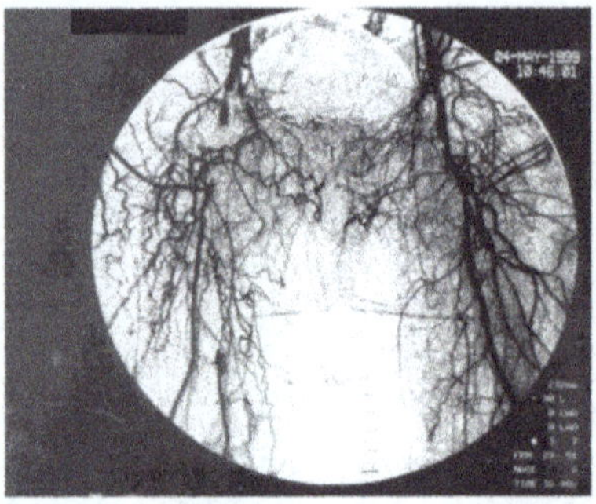

a

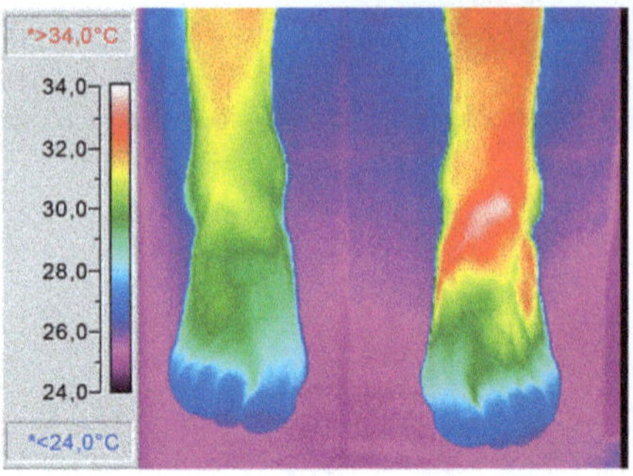

b

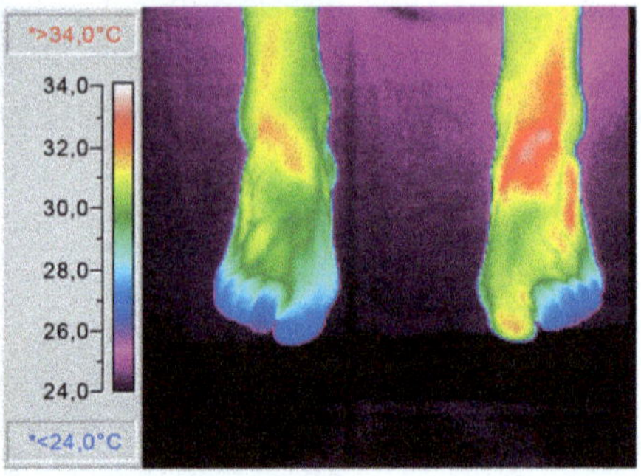

c

Figure 30.5. Arteriogram and thermograms of critical lower leg ischaemia, patient BS. (*a*) Arteriogram, before treatment, (*b*) thermogram, before treatment and (*c*) thermogram, after treatment with aloprostadilem (Prostavazin).

IOP Publishing

Infrared Imaging
A casebook in clinical medicine
Anna Jung, Janusz Żuber, Bolesław Kalicki, Wojciech Perdzyński, Marek Klewar and Piotr Murawski

Chapter 31

Infrared imaging of angiomatosis syndrome (Klippel–Trénaunay syndrome)

A 15-year-old girl attended the Children's Surgery Clinic, Military School of Medicine in Warsaw with angiomatosis of the right lower limb (Klippel–Trénaunay's syndrome). Large angiomas of the foot, calf (especially laterally), knee and thigh were assessed. These lesions were gradually becoming larger. In the thigh, angiomas present since late 1997 were inflamed with pain, fever, muscular contractions and difficulties in walking. The right mid-thigh circumference, measured standing, was 2.5 cm greater than the left mid-thigh. The upper right calf circumference was 3.5 cm greater than the upper left calf. There was 10° flexion deformity at the right knee joint. The right lower limb was 2 cm longer than the left lower limb. Doppler ultrasound examination of the right thigh confirmed an extensive venous angioma involving superficial and deep veins. Blood flow in these veins was evaluated in seated and supine positions. There was no evidence of thrombosis. An oscillating blood circulation was observed during the Valsalva manoeuvre and during compression. Blood flow within the angioma was not visualized. Cavernous angiomas were also examined in the foot and on the anterior and lateral surface of the thigh. In the left lower limb the popliteal vein and the long saphenous vein were narrower than the same veins in the left contralateral limb. The blood flow in the deep veins of the right lower limb was maintained but it was slower than in the lower left limb. There was normal blood flow in the arteries of both lower limbs. On venography, there was a conglomeration of dilated superficial veins. The deep venous system was not visualized, except for a portion of the popliteal vein. In surgery, very wide (2–2.5 cm) thin-walled angiomas were exposed and separated superficial to the fascia, with many connections between them and between the vessels situated sub-fascially. After ligation, the angiomas, which spread out in the upper calf, were

doi:10.1088/978-0-7503-1143-4ch31

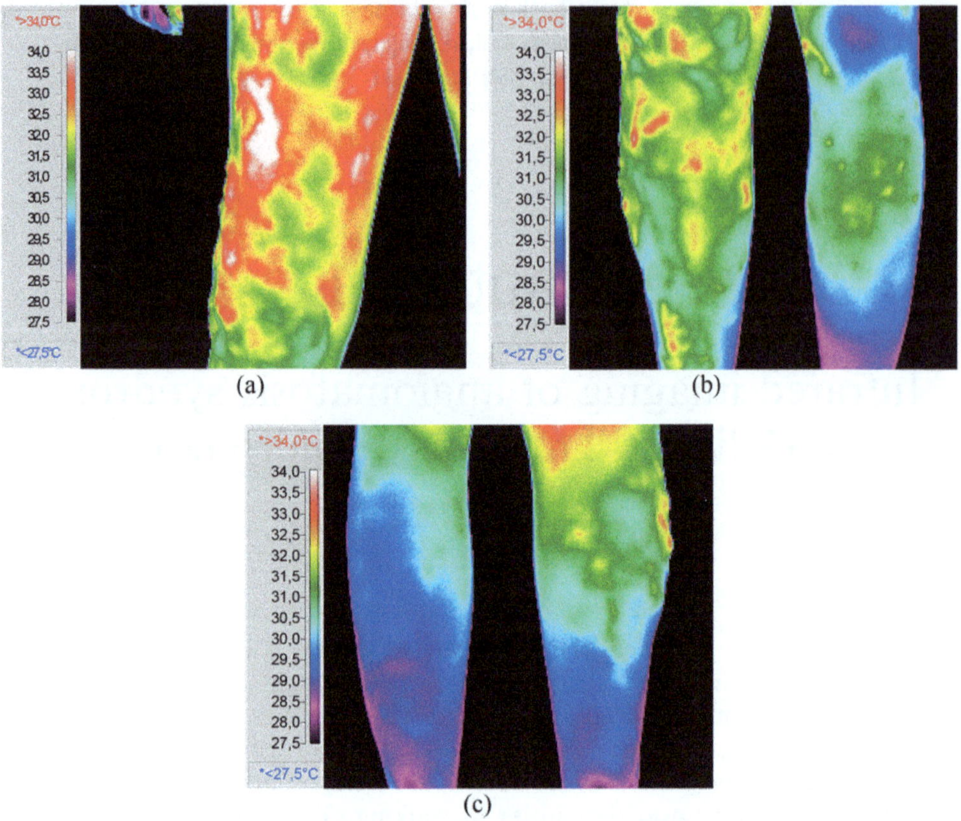

Figure 31.1. Thermograms of Klippel–Trénaunay (angiomatosis syndrome) in a 12-year-old girl (DA). The lower right extremity, before surgery. Temperature gradient: 4.5 °C. (*a*) Right upper leg, anterior view, (*b*) lower legs, anterior view and (*c*) lower legs, posterior view.

resealed. Post-operatively the wound healed well. Six months later there was no pain or inflammation in the calf.

On post-operative Doppler ultrasound there were no angiomas present in the operated area. The visualized blood flow through the popliteal vein and long saphenous vein was faster than before the operation but still slower than on the left side. Thermographic investigation of the right lower limb before the operation showed extensive hyperthermal areas in the right thigh, extending into the right popliteal and calf areas (figure 31.1). The hyperthermal areas corresponded to the images of conglomerates of dilated veins on the Doppler ultrasound (figure 31.2). Post-operatively, the areas of increased temperature were significantly smaller (figure 31.3). The temperature gradient between the area of abnormal veins and the surrounding tissue was about 4.5 °C pre-operatively, however, after the operation the gradient decreased to 2.5 °C. The thermographic visualization strictly correlated with the clinical assessment of the post-operative state.

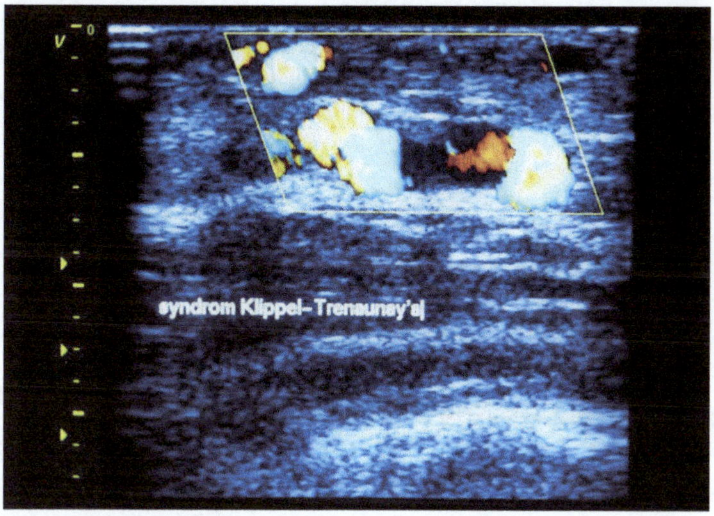

Figure 31.2. Post-operative Doppler ultrasound of Klippel–Trénaunay syndrome in a 12-year-old girl (DA).

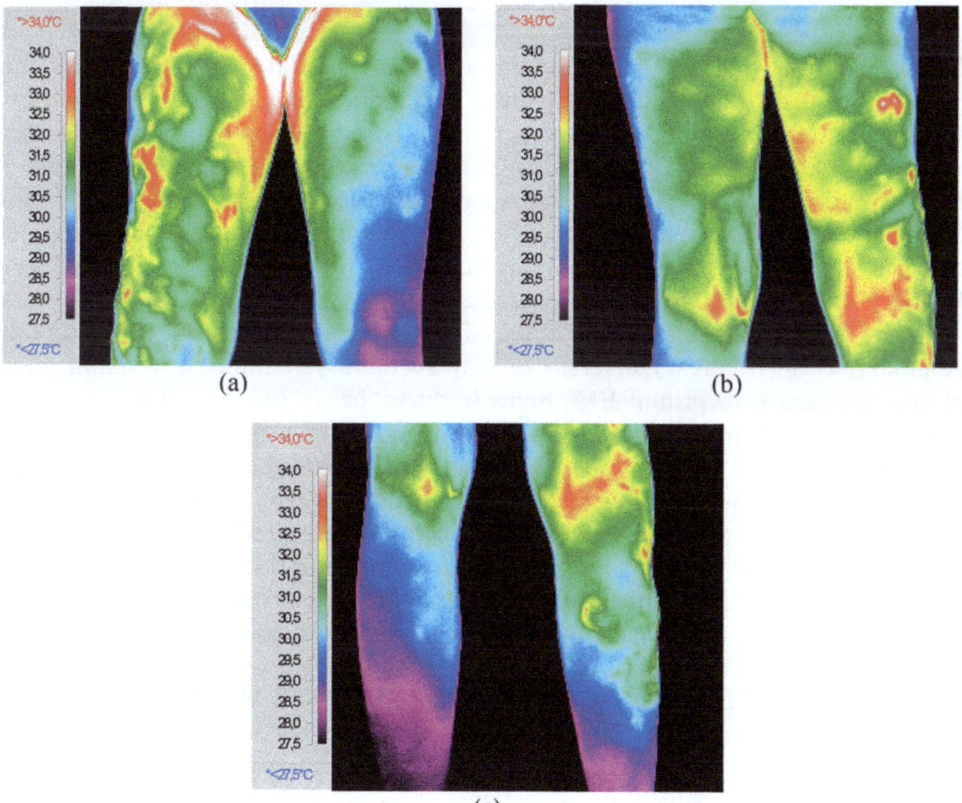

Figure 31.3. Thermograms of Klippel–Trénaunay syndrome in a 12-year-old girl (DA). Angiomatosis syndrome of the lower right extremity, after surgery. Temperature gradient: 2.5 °C. (*a*) Upper legs, anterior view, (*b*) upper legs, posterior view and (*c*) lower legs, posterior view.

IOP Publishing

Infrared Imaging
A casebook in clinical medicine
B Kalicki, A Jung, J Żuber, A Rustecka, A Lipińska-Opałka, B Nurowska-Wrzosek, Ł Gadomska vel Betka and Z Gaciong

Chapter 32

Thermal imaging: a monitoring tool for the treatment of erythromelalgia

Erythromelalgia (EM) is a rare condition (2.5–3.3/1000 000 yr^{-1}), with unexplained aetiology, with characteristic sudden onset with redness and limb inflammation with severe burning pain. Primary EM recognition is based only on clinical criteria, there are no characteristic histopathological changes or laboratory exam deviations. In EM symptoms have a recurrent character, most cases occur symmetrically, more often in the lower limb than the upper ones. Only cooling brings relief. The trophical changes (ulceration, necrosis) sometimes described are more likely to be the effect of frost-bite than evolution of the disease itself.

From August 2004 in the Clinic of Internal Diseases, Hypertension and Angiology of the Medical University of Warsaw there were multiple hospitalizations of two brothers with primal EM. Signs (redness, heavy feet and shank pain with characteristic burning and heat sensations) had been apparent in the younger brother (born 1986) since he was 13 years old. The older brother (born 1978) had felt the burning sensation in his lower limbs since he was six. Afterward redness and pain appeared. When he was 17 years old ulceration appeared in the area of his feet and toe deformation also appeared. Physical examination showed redness of the feet and the distal part of the shank and ulcerations of the toes. After receiving the results of additional tests the diagnosis of primary EM was confirmed. As treatment ranolazine was applied. The clinical effects of the treatment were monitored using an infrared camera (FLIR T-640), see figures 32.1 and 32.2. Analysis of the results showed no significant temperature differences in the areas of the body compared before and after treatment. The clinical assessment carried out by the attending physician and the assessment of the patients' drug administration did not show any significant improvement.

doi:10.1088/978-0-7503-1143-4ch32

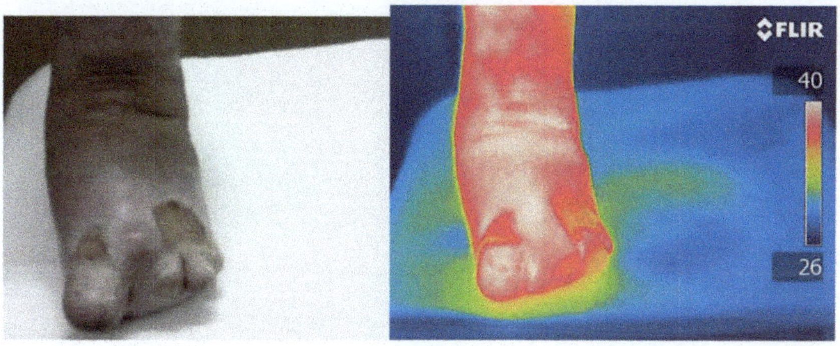

(a) (b)

Figure 32.1. Photo (*a*) and thermographic image (*b*) of the left foot of the elder brother.

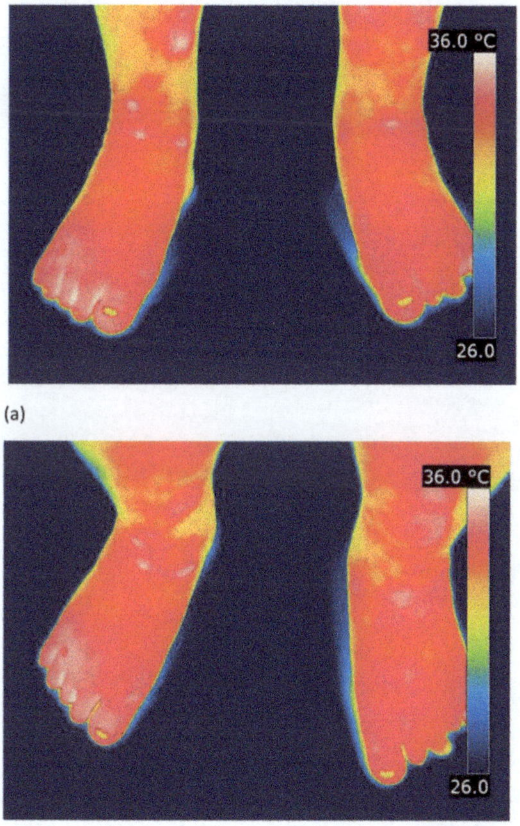

(b)

Figure 32.2. Thermograms of the younger brother's feet before (*a*) and after the treatment (*b*).

Lightning Source UK Ltd.
Milton Keynes UK
UKHW050620060821
388415UK00003B/64

9 780750 311441